You Mean, Besides the Cancer?

A CAREGIVER'S JOURNEY —
SOME DAYS THE CANCER WAS THE
LEAST OF OUR WORRIES

BY BOB MARCOTTE

Copyright © 2012 by Bob Marcotte
First Edition – February 2012

Cover design by Brad Boling

All photography copyright © Bob Marcotte except where otherwise credited.

ISBN
978-1-77097-198-1 (Hardcover)
978-1-77097-199-8 (Paperback)
978-1-77097-200-1 (eBook)

All rights reserved.

No part of this publication may be reproduced in any form, or by any means, electronic or mechanical, including photocopying, recording, or any information browsing, storage, or retrieval system, without permission in writing from the publisher.

Published by:

FriesenPress
Suite 300 – 852 Fort Street
Victoria, BC, Canada V8W 1H8

www.friesenpress.com

Distributed to the trade by The Ingram Book Company

For information on bulk orders contact:
info@friesenpress.com or fax 1-888-376-7026

Table of Contents

Prologue x
Chronology of Medical Events xi
The Lobbyists 1
A Breath Before Battle 3
Et Homo Factus Est 5
Time and Tide 9
What Cancer Looks Like 10
In the Beginning Was the Word 14
A Change of Identity 16
Rest is a Weapon 17
Now the fun really begins 19
We're going to Stanford 20
The Quality of Mercy 21
Advocate of Angels 23
Can You Hear Me Now? 26
Sometimes she cries 30
Pain, in its many forms 31
Graceland for the Gaseous 34
You mean, besides the cancer? 37
Pre-school 40
Droppin' Dimes 42
Laps 45
A Fog, Only Less 49
I make this look good 53
The Beach 54
A Question of God 56
Vacancy 59
Optimism and Fatigue 61
Hell On Wheels 64
The Way We Were 65
Sisyphus Meet Icarus 67

Fruitful Absurdity	69
Quantum Uncertainty	71
The Road Ahead	73
Today, Tomorrow, Friday, Forever	74
Playdays	80
Because	82
Conversations	83
Shopping for Joy	85
IF	87
Waiting Redefined	88
Final Approach	92
Surgery Day	94
The Walking Tour of Hell – Part 1	95
The Walking Tour of Hell – Part 2	101
Intermission	107
Another "M" Word	109
Stairway to Heaven	112
Passing Through	113
Lucky Dog	116
It's nothing to worry about, it's only pain.	120
Good News, Bad News	122
Tough News	123
Pass the Matches	124
A Matter of Time	126
F Words	127
Welcome to the block, Homo-Erectus	129
Tonight, she healed me	131
Stand Up, Stand Down	133
Graduation Day	136
The Art of Survival	138
I Never Wanted A Tat	140
Epilogue	141
Add Your Voice	142

For Carole,

I know you say that I didn't "sign up for this", but I did, the first time I told you I love you.

Still do,
Bob

*The quality of mercy is not strain'd,
It droppeth as the gentle rain from heaven
Upon the place beneath. It is twice blest:
It blesseth him that gives and him that takes.*

The Merchant Of Venice Act 4, scene 1, 180–187

> I would thank you from the bottom of my heart,
> but for you my heart has no bottom.
>
> -Author Unknown

This is where an author usually thanks people for their help with the book. In this case, we have to thank people for our survival. Literally, without them, my wife would be gone.

That thought still scares me. It's humbling to think that there are people out there who will do *anything* to help you during a time like we endured.

To Mary Smith, R.N, F.N.P, M.S.N. and her medical friends who so gracefully gave of their time to teach me what the test results meant and what questions to ask our doctors;

To Dr. Dina Ibrahim, our local medical oncologist who led us to Stanford and still continues to care for Carole;

To all the medical magicians and staff at Stanford, especially Dr. Dan Chang who, as excellent a radiologist as he is, had the humility to seek alternative treatments when his treatment options left him unsatisfied, and that led us to…

Dr. Stefan Mindea, the neurosurgeon who led the surgical teams over the 29 hours my wife spent on the operating table but, more importantly, when we knew we had no choice, Dr. Mindea's excellence, honesty and integrity made us believe we were never without hope.

Sincere thanks to our family and friends who supported us with love and prayers. We could not have borne this weight without your help.

To Kathy Hamlin, for organizing all the care giving, and always with a smile;

To Christine Lindley, for just being Christine Lindley, that was always perfect and welcome in itself;

To Carole's sister Susan, for putting your life on hold for a few weeks to help us organize ours;

To the Boling family who adopted us and treated us like family from day one and who still do;

And to Rick and Denise: you have the soot of hell on your shoes, just like we do, because you followed us everywhere we had to go. You propped us up when we faltered, caught us when we fell, and the scary part is that you'd do it all again, all out of love. We love you, too. Thank you.

And to Carole's Mom, you gave birth to one tough girl! And thank *YOU* for that – and so much more!

Prologue

I will start this book with an absolute truth.

Being a Caregiver is the most intense, thankless and painful job on earth.

You have the honor of a front row seat to your loved one's pain and decline. Often this is your only perk, and to earn it you have to deal with an army of medical professionals who often have lost their ability to feel or the energy to care, unless YOU engage them and invite them to be a part of the solution.

You also have to deal with well meaning family and friends who unintentionally complicate things with ideas, opinions, and sometimes actions that in the end only hurt. These are tender situations and require great patience. Often, they are in a panic, more so than you, and are desperate to do "something", even if that something wastes time and burns up your precious energy.

Have faith in yourself, you can do this, and hopefully this book can shortcut the learning curve that sliced me to shreds.

Eventually, you will grow into something indestructible, someone who no longer feels pain, who no longer needs sleep, and will do absolutely anything for your spouse's care and comfort. I know that sounds horrible, but it sometimes becomes necessary.

From what I've read, women fall into this job more naturally than men. I'm not an expert on that, but I can say this book was written by a man, and from a man's perspective. Sometimes that means impatience, anger, and colorful words from my Navy days. I promise you, any rough language is not used for dramatic effect; it was exactly what I was feeling at the time and still the most honest and eloquent language I know.

And a few words about the photography — most of the images are mine. It seems like a different life ago when I took pictures that did not relate to medicine or tears. I could have easily doubled the size of this book by taking more pictures at the most intimate and difficult of times, but I did not want to invade my wife's privacy, or mine. The intensity of those seconds will never be forgotten by either of us, and most likely never shared with anyone else.

And, believe it or not, the time frame for this book is January 4th to April 28th, 2011.

Yeah, I can't believe it either.

Chronology of Medical Events

2003 – Carole was diagnosed with mucinous cystadenoma. Though not technically cancer, it is known to create huge tumors which require surgical removal. Pathology on mucinous cystadenoma typically comes back as inconclusive for cancer. This tumor is no different.

2006 – Another significant tumor requiring surgery was found. Pathology on this tumor is inconclusive for cancer.

2010 – In October of 2010, Carole was complaining of a backache. Eventually, she had an MRI of her lumbar spine which showed no bulging disc as suspected, but rather a huge mass in her pelvis.

On December 10th, 2010 Carole had her third surgery to remove this latest mass. The pathology continued to be inconclusive for cancer, but it was clear that whatever this was had morphed into a far more aggressive form.

In late December we met the Oncologist for the first time and she sent us for further testing.

Our first test was scheduled for January 4, 2011.

The book starts there.

The Lobbyists

January 4, 2011

The building is modern; the staff is so young that the magazines in the lobby seem older than they are. Their smiles are perfect and the service impeccable. The only downside in all this designer beauty is the clientele.

The people who pass through these doors are all on their way to the pearly gates, as we all are, but this clientele is taking the Express.

Cancer, other diseases no one can spell, and bad luck fill the waiting rooms. While the perfect, youthful staff have yet to experience their first wrinkle, this clientele wait with wrinkled brows. Unspoken concern is the silent topic of conversation between strangers who now have so much in common.

There appear to be three strata of life in the lobby. The televisions quietly remind all who look of the perfection demanded by our culture, the culture of beauty and youth. The commercials constantly reinforce your flaws. Buy make up, lose weight, get rich, drive this car and you'll be culturally vital, you'll be relevant.

The staff, who appear to be getting younger by the hour, look up and soak in the future of their beliefs. They share a morning breakfast of fresh fruit. They discuss last night's work out and their plans for the weekend. Even new eyeglass frames on a staff member bring the welcoming machine to a halt as an informal staff meeting is called to compliment the wearer. Yes, these beautiful ones never consider life on the other side of the reception desk. They empathize in the most attractive and professional of ways, but they don't ever imagine themselves among the clientele, except for helping with paperwork, of course.

And then there are the wrinkled ones, wrinkled by time or worry, or both. This group seldom glances up to see the perfect world. Their energy is being consumed, as well as their bodies, by insecurity; by challenge and fear; by mortality and denial. And paperwork.

And they sit in silence with so much in common. They have all waited for a similar stranger to pronounce the state of their health, to predict the length and quality of their future. They all sit in the same meditation, the same silent meditation.

And there are so many insults to be endured as they silently sit in the lobby. They're taken in the "order received". They need "authorization" to be treated. Their pain is "managed", and only by appointment. The perfect ones politely turn away and pretend not to notice the hair loss, the bandages from surgery, the scars of battle. Or battles.

Not only are the lobby sitters unlucky and diseased, they also drift further and further away from the perfect TV world. There is no makeup that covers pain. There is no value in this culture to being bald and scarred unless you're a celebrity. In that rare case, you are a trend-setter, a trail blazer, a talent, someone to emulate. No one emulates the lobbyists.

And the lobby continues to fill and empty, like the belly of a beast. The doors appear to be alive, swallowing the diseased, culturally irrelevant like a dragon. Each step taken is a step closer to being swallowed whole. Whole lives, memories and dreams included.

And the beast continues feeding, every new door triggers the beast's appetite, more doors, more whole lives.

And so much silence. So much in common, so much silence.

A Breath Before Battle

January 6, 2011

If everyone's life is a book, and every day a page, then there are some days that deserve to be dog-eared. Your high school graduation, your wedding day, the birth of your children, and the day that your doctor discusses chemotherapy with you for the first time.

Yes, we saw the pathology report. Yes, we expected a 'next step', but chemo? In my layman's mind, isn't that what desperate people keep as a last resort to save their lives? (And isn't it ironic that it's referred to as a last 'resort', as if you exhausted all the other beach-side, four-star hotels and now you're stuck staying at **Motel 6**, but at least they kept the light on for you?).

No, this is not that resort. It's the resort where they surgically implant a "port" into you, so the chemicals designed to kill cancer can flow through you without obstruction. The chemicals designed to kill fast-growing cells like your hair, like the inside of your mouth, like the stuff causing immeasurable pain.

The return on this investment could be huge. Kill cancer and continue to live. Sounds like a winning lottery ticket – except for the nausea, the vomiting, the mouth sores, and the hair loss.

Our culture looks down on the unattractive. A treatment of chemo is almost like being thrown outside the city walls in ancient times. You are a leper, you are misunderstood, show yourself to the rabbi before being considered "clean", before returning to society, lest ye upset the popular concept of beauty.

Today, I am not the one to receive the chemo blessing from the oncologist, it is my dear wife. But someday, if given that same pronouncement, my intent would be to walk tall and proudly among the ignoring masses, showing them that the struggle for life is at least as beautiful as "life as we know it".

In this small but battle-tested family, we celebrate the victories, as small as they may be, and the mercies, as rare as they may be. My wife may need to wear a scarf. She may even decide to wear a wig, but her struggle and ultimate victory makes her someone I want to be near. Anyone can watch TV and see the car they need to drive, the makeup that covers unsightly blemishes, and the mutual fund that will make them rich, but how many people do you know who realize the value of every second? A life threatened is a life magnified. We will amplify every moment into a moment worth remembering, a memory, a bookmark.

Today, I pity those who casually see tomorrow as a birthright, what many just call 'another day'.

Tomorrow for us is another celebration of life.

We don't hold fast to the "another day" premise, and because of that, life has become more pure, more worthy, and more worth living.

Et Homo Factus Est

January 8, 2011

The question constantly dangling before my artsy-fartsy, philosophical mind is the meaning, quality and length of human life. This is obviously motivated by my wife's diagnosis and projected chemo treatment path.

And, just as a matter of business, I will admit that I write now to vent, to rant, to let the frustration out. In return, I've gotten some very supportive and thoughtful feedback from friends and family.

Speaking of feedback, I have heard from more than one friend saying that a diagnosis that requires chemo is not the death sentence it once was. They point out people in their lives who have beaten this disease and are living whole lives again. Yes, I realize that, but never has one so dear to me been so threatened in my adult life.

And never have I felt so helpless.
Lord, what is man that you should care for him?...Psalm 144

Ironically, I have **NOT** heard many asking why there is no mention of God in these recent posts. Honestly, I don't really know. Perhaps it's the fact that I'm still in shock, perhaps it's the "boots on the ground" approach I am taking with this, that if it has to get done, then I'll do it. Quite honestly, until recently when Carole's pain was finally starting to get managed, it was pure exhaustion that stopped me from considering anything that was not immediate or practical.

I have played over a million notes on the piano trying in vain to describe God. I also admit to never having found a perfect theology to explain God.

God, to be sure, I know you are there, but I often doubt that you know I'm here. I know that I am wholly imperfect, but I also know I've tried to live a life that honors you more than offends you. I have searched and found clues, circumstantial evidence, small tracks in the snow, but nothing that makes me feel as if I am on the right trail. Honestly, we need far more help down here than we're getting. We need far more insight into the grand plan if we're going to be part of it.

ET HOMO FACTUS EST

This has led me to a completely Bob-like, off-the-wall thought that should surprise no one who knows me.

Perhaps the meaning of this struggle, of all this misery and mystery is to demonstrate to people what it is to be fully human. I'm not claiming to have had conversations with burning bushes recently, but the only single thing all people on earth have in common is that they are people, and people have demonstrated a determined commonality in being born, living, and dying.

In between the being born part and dying part is a long, painful struggle to survive, to find an identity, to find meaning and perhaps even influence this life in some positive way. And for most of us, all this effort ends in futility. We chase earthly shadows, like trying to be the next Ansel Adams, but how badly would the world have been affected if there never had been an Ansel Adams? We chase what fulfills us, but is that truly the meaning of this existence?

THE POWER OF DISTRACTION

I believe that all people are wired to worship. I also believe that if this life were as whizz-bang fulfilling as we think it should be, then there would be no need for distraction.

Let me clarify here, when I refer to distraction, I do not refer to the arts. The arts are humankind's way of holding a mirror before itself, allowing each person to judge whether or not they see themselves, and whether they want to be a part of what they see. And the arts are also far more eloquent than the typical person can be. Think of it this way: **where words fail, music begins**.

No, when I say distraction, I am referring to the pop-culture, slickly marketed crap that comes from the bowels of our culture, typically from a zip code of 90210, the "entertainment" with no artistic value except for gun battles and boobies. I have more respect for a porn flick than much of what is poured into the eyes and ears of people from "entertainers". How many people have you seen killed on TV or in the movies? How many "imaginative" ways did they die? Guns, cars, chain saws, drowning, etc., you name it and you've either seen it yourself or heard about it. No, this is not art. It is a pointless attempt to distract people from their everyday lives, take them out of their existence and put them in someone else's for a short time.

And this is what people worship. They worship the "musicians", "actors" and "celebrities" (those who have even less talent than "musicians" and "actors"). They worship the violence; they worship the explosions; the noise; the distraction. And at the end of all these countless hours of watching what they worship, are they any better? Have they improved? Have they evolved?

Recently, I sat through a movie called "The Expendables". It had no story to speak of, just muscles and bombs and guns and blood. It was a waste of two hours of my life and had no value. I fully expect a sequel.

THE POWER OF COMPASSION

How does this rant against distraction work its way into a post about God? Perhaps because what we worship often shapes our expectations. It's not out of the question to think that some people believe that the Second Coming will be the most enormous hi-def, 3D, iMax, surround sound event the world has ever seen, with a soundtrack to die for. And the clothes will be **fabulous** (of course)!

Since my wife has fallen ill, I have been asking God for a miracle, a **BIG** miracle, some different test results, some new painless treatment, the 'cure of all cures'.

For the record, I am still waiting for the big miracle, but I have been moved daily by the small miracles around me, namely the care and compassion people have shown for her, and for me. And believe me, ***this compassion has power***.

Like the people who have taken considerable time out of their lives to cook dinners for us.

Or the friends who are medical professionals, who have taken even more time patiently explaining to us what is happening, what the reports mean, what the future may hold. And their standing offer to call anytime, 24/7, if they can be of help is **sincere.** I know, because I recently took someone up on her offer, and she was here in minutes.

And how about the pharmacy techs who ask about my wife every time I get a script filled? And how my script is always ready, no matter how few minutes ago it was called in?

And how about the people I work for and with? They tell me to take what time I need, my wife comes first. In a profit-driven culture, my wife suddenly comes first.

And how about my two buddies, both with pony tails (yes, I'm envious) who check in on me? They keep holding me up when I very much want to fall down.

And how about the nurses and doctors who **actually care**? Yes, they do their jobs with professional efficiency, but only they can **decide to care**.

And how about our three dogs and one cat who sense that Carole is ill and surround her, guard her, will her to recovery? They are "only" animals, but they know. And they very much care.

Any single act of compassion does not seem remarkable by itself, but added together, this compassion is very powerful.

Life changing actually.

THIS IS NOT A SPOILER ALERT

No, I don't have any answers. I can't ruin all your fun by telling you how all this will end, but I was led to another question by all this. Think of it as a perspective check for all of us, because otherwise it won't work.

(And please don't think that I am recruiting here. My question applies to you regardless of whether or not you follow an organized religion, whether you're a "free agent" waiting for some impressive theology to explain everything, or whether you just consider yourself "spiritual".)

What if all this compassion being spilled over my family is not a clue that God exists, or even a sign from God, but IS God?

What if God's power is so vast, that he could make a difference with a whisper, rather than a Second Coming? No sunbeams breaking through the clouds, no earthquakes, no lighting, no floods (sorry Hollywood), just a whisper from His lips to your ear that someone needs you. Someone needs help and He has chosen you, and only you can do it perfectly.

What if our purpose is not wrapped up in professional or personal achievement, but in simple human compassion?

This idea would certainly address why there is pain and suffering in this world. It's there to give us an opportunity to give compassionate care to those who need it, and in doing so, unleash a little more God into the world. No one single act, but countless acts. You can change lives that way. You can change worlds that way.

But it's a conscious decision on a person's part. Each person can choose to be compassionate or simply walk away. No, your one simple little act of compassion won't change the world, but billions of simple little acts of compassion unleashed every minute is probably best described as a **BIG** miracle, wouldn't you agree?

I'VE USED UP ALL MY BIG WORDS...

Walking through this life as a compassionate human being is a risk. There will be times when your compassion goes unnoticed or even unwelcome. But if that decision is truly yours, what would you prefer to do, unleash God or unleash hell?

And in that moment of decision, perhaps you'll hear a whisper that makes you feel a little less alone.

Time and Tide

January 9, 2011

The pause, the calm before the storm, the wait.

These days, time seems to have stopped. Pain is "controlled" as best as it can be, but life is anything but controlled. Speculation continues, and fear rises and falls like a tide. We cannot control the tide, it controls us, and we react to its rise and fall. Speculation and ignorance are the enemies now.

At a time of struggle or stress, most people reach back to what they "know", what they are most comfortable with. Here's mine, and in my opinion, these are some of the most eloquent words ever written.

Keep watch, dear Lord, with those who work, or watch, or weep this night, and give your angels charge over those who sleep.

Tend the sick, Lord Christ; give rest to the weary, bless the dying, soothe the suffering, pity the afflicted, shield the joyous; and all for your love's sake. Amen.

From the night service of Compline, The Book of Common Prayer 1979
(Episcopal Book of Common Prayer, page 124)

'nuff said.

What Cancer Looks Like

January 10, 2011

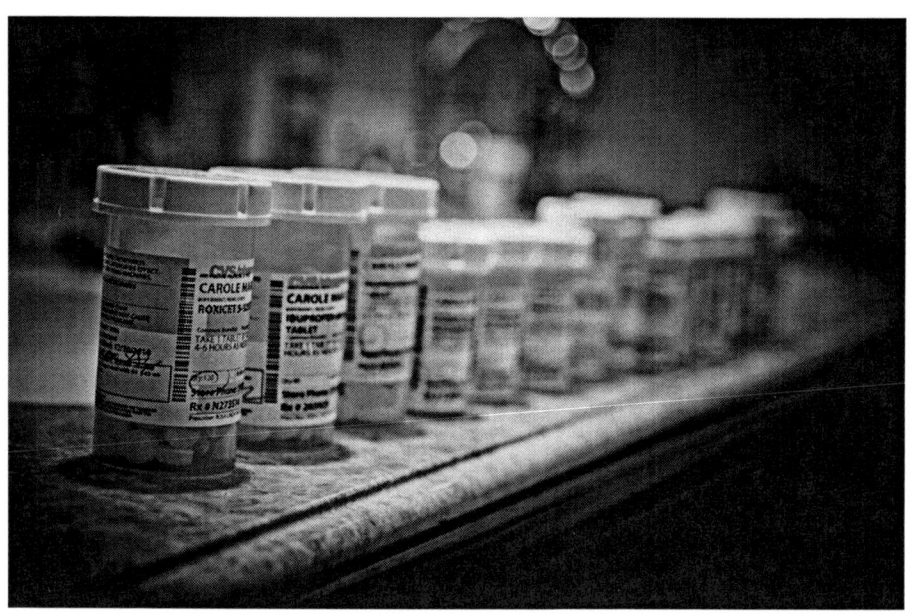

So many bottles…

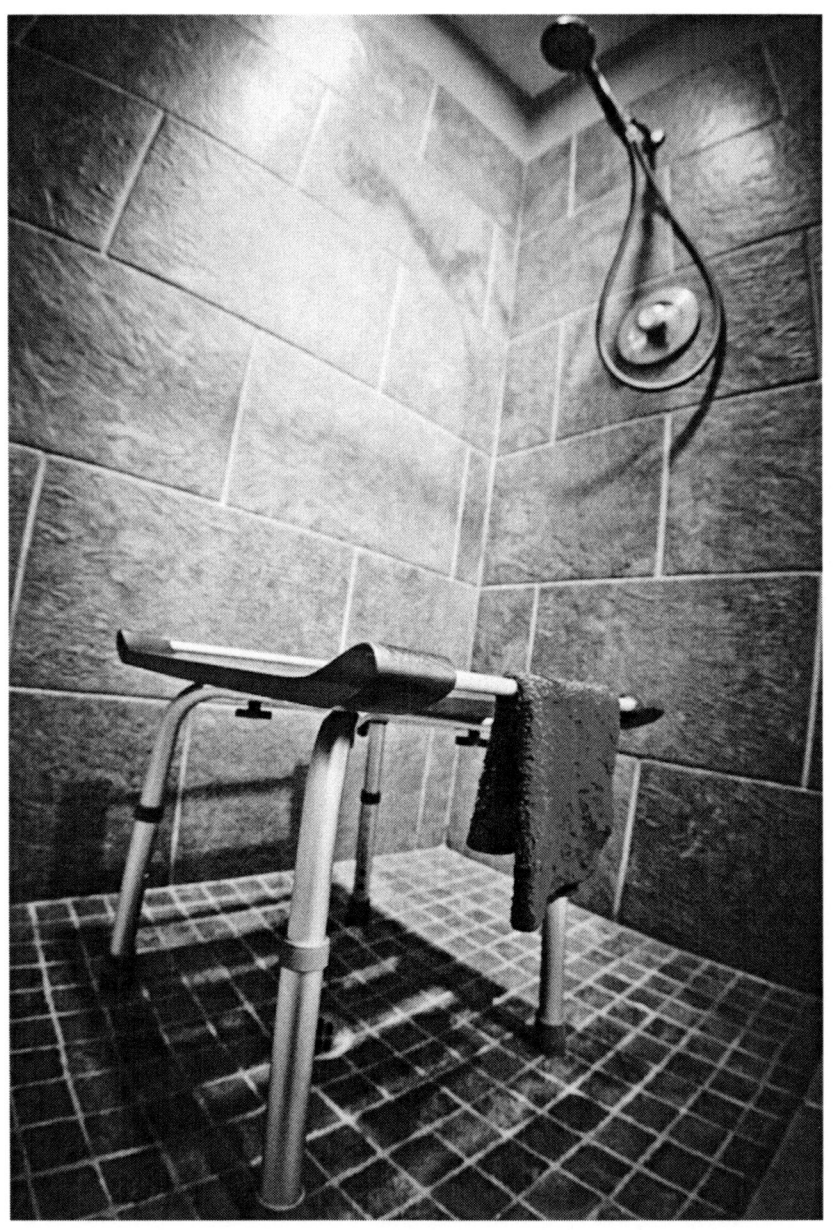
She can no longer stand in the shower.

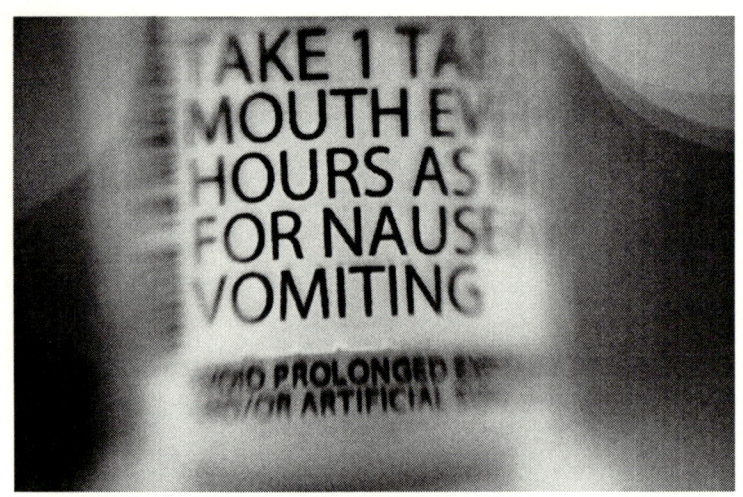

Some days it works, some days...not so much.

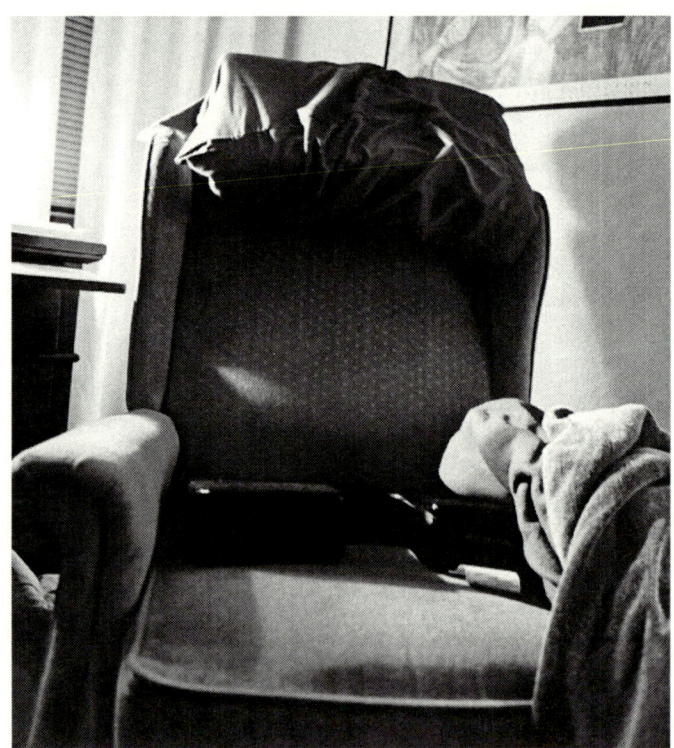

Her Most Comfortable Spot

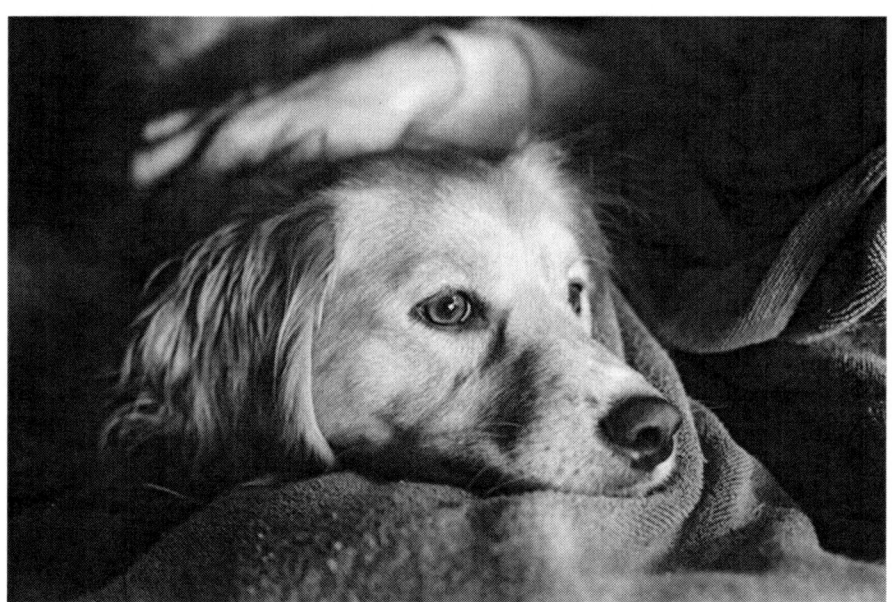

Her Constant Companion

In the Beginning Was the Word

January 10, 2011

...and the word was cancer.

Ironic. John starts his gospel at the beginning of time. Our doctor uttered that word and suddenly time, at least for us, started over. The Big Bang.

There is no mention of "last summer", "first date", "three day weekend", just time before the diagnosis and time since. BC and AD. Before Cancer. After Diagnosis.

And time has made a mockery of us with this.

Waiting is so much longer and more difficult. Waiting for the pain meds to kick in is eternal. The time watching your wife waiting for the pain meds to kick in has not yet been defined in my language, but it's far beyond eternal.

We need new words to describe the time spent fasting before a procedure, the time waiting for results, the way the night moves so slowly now, and how quickly time passes just before the alarm goes off.

A Little Known Fact

I work in a building filled with supermodels. Yes, it's true, but I'm only talking about the women.

I think of three of these remarkable women right now. They are not remarkable for their beauty alone, they all have intelligence, integrity and soul. Your mother would have hit you with her car had you broken up with any of these women. (In fact, she would have run over you twice if she could drive a stick.)

One is recently married, one is recently engaged, and one just today had the youngest of her two beautiful daughters start pre-school. Each is on a different place on the path, but all have something in common. Time will fly by.

They will look up at some point and ask, "Where did the time go?" Someday they will look behind them and see intentionally crafted, wonderful lives. Beautiful lives.

My wife does not work in my building, but she is very much like these women. She has improved life every place she has stood on this planet, and yet here we are. Winners (or losers) of a genetic disease lotto, caught in a time trap, trying to come to grips with a life that is now unintentionally crafted, far from wonderful and intensely ugly at times. A life undeserved in every respect.

A LIFE SLOWED DOWN

Words such as chemo, port, second opinion, prescription...pain...all resonate in our minds with little to stop them, as we wait for an appointment or an "opinion". And all these big words resonate loudly while other words are mute, like assurance, guarantee, comfort, peace. Those are words seldom used to describe life, even less so now.

Cancer is really more like ten thousand paper cuts than a single disease. No one cut will kill you, but the constant stream of indignities and diagnosis really takes its toll, perhaps none more that the slowing of time. While I wish my supermodel friends all the joy a person can hold, I wish THEY could experience time like we do. Where every second is not so much lived as absorbed.

And I hope they never have to endure the cruel joke that time has played on us.

A Change of Identity

January 11, 2011

Carole had her 'port' surgically implanted today. This allows the medical types to deliver the chemo directly into a major vein near her heart. It speeds the delivery of **LOTS** of stuff that no one should ever have to endure.

Whether you see chemo patients as victims or heroes, she's one of ***'them'*** now.

Rest is a Weapon

January 12, 2011

Sadly, today was actually just another day.

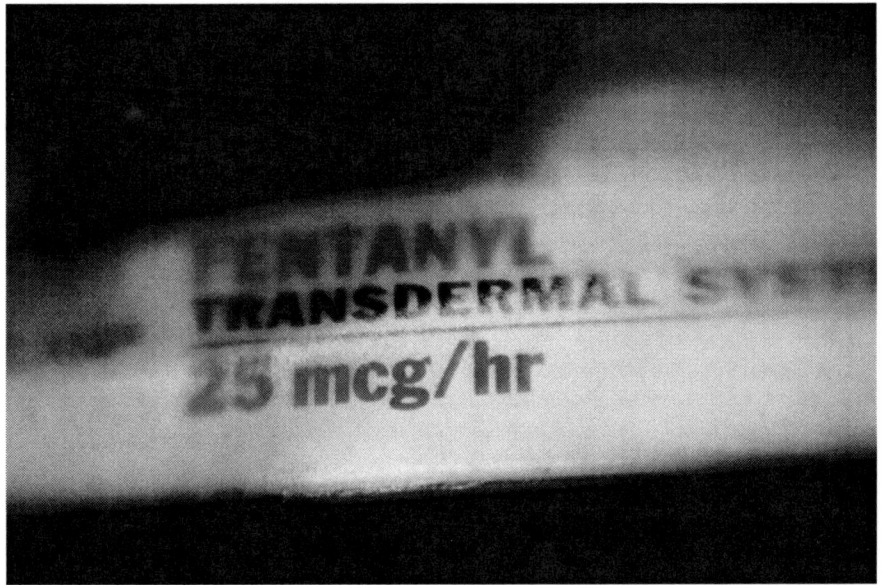

Neither of us slept well. In fact, I slept on the floor next to our bed.

She doesn't breathe anymore, she sighs. She moans under her breath while she naps. She suffers.

Today, coffee revived me, but anger motivated me. We had an appointment with the oncologist and I wanted relief for Carole, relief for me, even if I pissed off the doc.

The drive there was mostly wordless. No trying to make her smile. The laugh lines I once studied on her sleeping face are hardly used any more.

She moans again.

And while we drive, I sense a change in me. I am so exhausted by all this that I sometimes stop watching and listening. How could my wife's suffering be demoted to background noise? It's not; it never was, but sometimes....

OPEN BAR

I have my checklist ready for the oncologist; I even wrote it down. The Doc enters and quickly agrees with everything I ask for, including doubling Carole's pain meds. I was too tired to be suspicious and then she tells us why.

The cancer is in the bone, the most painful cancer there is. My wife has open bar at the pharmacy; the doc will write as many scripts as needed to make her comfortable.

I have been punched so often with tough news lately that I actually thought that, intellectually, I could shake this one off, but emotionally I was dropped to my knees. In the bone.

IN the bone.

DOUBLE DOWN

We went to the pharmacy with a fist full of scripts, and then home. There, while she was lying on the couch, unable to find comfort, I made a decision. *Fuck it.*

On went **TWO** pain patches at the same time followed by **TWO** pain pills thirty minutes later. Dammit, we need to get on top of this agony once and for all, her suffering has been too long and it **WILL** end now. We'll worry about side effects if they crop up. We'll wake doctors in **THEIR** sleep if we have to, but we're providing rest for this woman if I have to wake up the whole world.

Two hours later she tells me she's feeling better. When I came back from my second job, she tells me she's feeling even better than when I left. Sleep may happen tonight, a pause in her suffering. I thanked Jesus for this little miracle so elusive. I'm sure I'll be asking for more miracles in the future.

THE FIGHT DOES NOT BEGIN SOON ENOUGH

The doc already had sent slides of Carole's tumor to Stanford for a second opinion. Today, she agreed to send Carole. An **ASAP** consult may take Stanford weeks or even months to address, but the doc also agreed not to postpone chemo while waiting for them. Chemo will start as soon as the second pathology report comes back, tentatively scheduled for the week of my birthday. I could care less about that. The only gift I want is the opportunity to start fighting this cowardly bastard hiding somewhere inside my wife. I know it will put her through hell, but I will drag her through it if needed. We'll buy postcards and take tourist pictures, but we are not stopping in hell, we're just passing through. The tumor will be staying in hell. This tumor will die.

Until then, rest is a weapon. I will help her rest and eat and gain strength.

Then, it's game time.

Now the Fun Really Begins

January 13, 2011

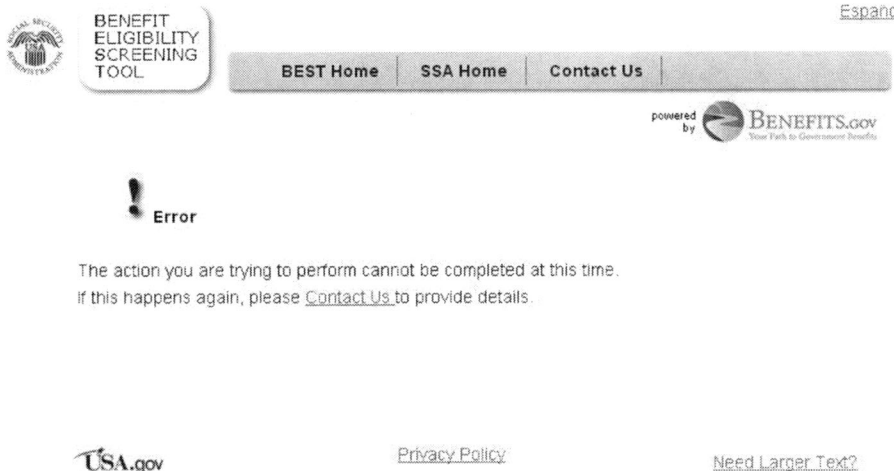

The beautiful graphic you see above is brought to you by the United Stated Social Security Administration. This was the result of using their online Benefit Eligibility Screening Tool to determine which, if any, benefits Carole may be eligible for.

Preceeding this magic moment was a ten-plus minute phone call of negotiating voice menus, attempting to speak to someone at the California Employment Development Department about Paid Family Leave.

I was handed a brochure by the woman who runs the Human Resource department here at work. The brochure lists **EIGHT** different phone numbers to call so you can speak with someone about Paid Family Leave in the language you are most comfortable with. The options are English, Espanol, Cantonese, Vietnamese, Armenian, Punjabi, Tagalog, and TTY for the hearing impaired.

At the end of my wait, I was rewarded with the following message:

The maximum number of callers has been reached, please call again.

The message comes through loud and clear in any language. This is **not** going to be easy.

We're going to Stanford

January 13, 2011

Our oncologist managed to get us an appointment at the Stanford Cancer Center on the 26th. Everything is on hold until after the results are back.

The Quality of Mercy

January 15, 2011

> The quality of mercy is not strain'd,
> It droppeth as the gentle rain from heaven
> Upon the place beneath. It is twice blest:
> It blesseth him that gives and him that takes.
> *'The Merchant of Venice' ~ Shakespeare*

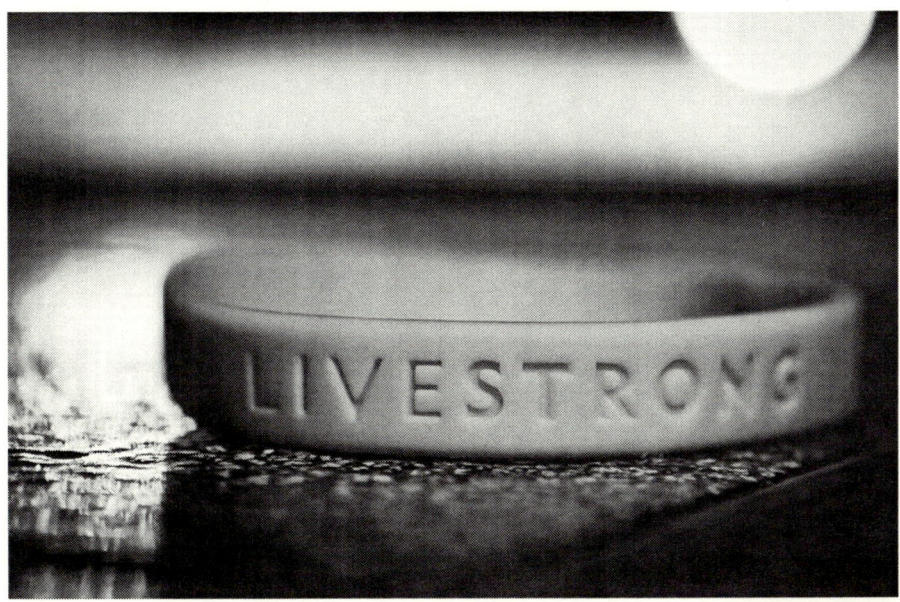

Cancer is a curse, I have no doubt about that, but if there is such a thing as balance in 'life,' then the curse is balanced by compassion. Compassion does not get the headlines it deserves. Compassion is silent, overlooked and often assumed. "Someone else" often takes care of "them".

Since it has been our turn to be "them", we are humbled by the compassion being shown to us on a daily basis. Tonight, we dined on chicken pot pies given to us by a co-worker and his wife. Yesterday, two co-workers put in their own time and effort to find nausea options for Carole (and provided samples).

As I type this, Mom-in-law is out having dinner and seeing a movie with a friend who volunteered, unrequested.

This is by no means a complete list. In fact, it's not even a complete list over the last 48 hours.

If compassion is the result of a whisper from God into one person's ear, then our lives are a living example that God does LOTS of whispering. Every hour, every day, another whisper.

There are few guarantees about how all this will end, except that I will fight for Carole until my last breath, and that the compassion we're being shown will continue, and continue, and continue.

Thank you God.
Thank you friends.
You make us stronger.
Your whispers are deafening.

Advocate of Angels

January 15, 2011

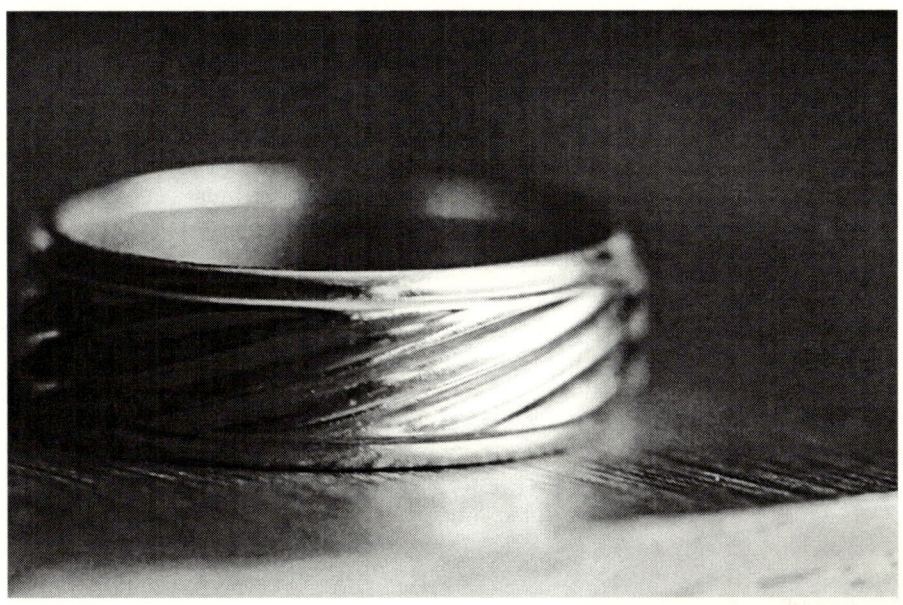

(A caregiver's cheat sheet)

I was motivated to put together a cheat sheet on some things I have recently been forced to learn. I don't know how useful this will be, but here are my thoughts, in no particular order. And keep in mind that this is a man's view, so feelings are sometimes optional.

I honestly don't know how some people do this alone. I truly believe that people can die from falling into the cracks. As well-intentioned as our doctors, nurses and medical institutions are, there are wide cracks that patients can fall into where they suffer in some lonely solitude, waiting for a phone call or a prescription from an overloaded medical professional who, in their own human frailty, forgot, or never wrote.

I function as Carole's advocate. I force communication between doctors. I build a team. Receptionists know my name. Pharmacists and their staff ask how Carole is when I pick up scripts. Even nurses, technicians, on-call doctors, nurses' aides, anyone who becomes a part of Carole's care for more than a few minutes is brought up to speed, and is made to feel a part of the treatment. There is no one of insignificance in my wife's treatment. I try to show respect for their expertise, and in return I get their best efforts.

You have to have mercy on doctors. They've spent 12 years of their lives in school getting an MD. As much as they may have a compassionate world view, they only know **what** they treat, not **who** they treat. It is up to you to teach them. Speak for your spouse. You'd be surprised at how stoic some people get in front of a medical professional. Tell the doc what **YOU** saw and **HOW** she really felt. In many cases, it's the only honest thing the doc hears in the appointment, especially early in the diagnosis stage.

Guys, when you married your spouse, you didn't just take her hand in marriage, you got her whole Barbie collection. There is the Happy Spouse Barbie, the Angry Spouse Barbie, the Shy Spouse Barbie, the I Want to Fight Barbie, the I'm Ready to Kiss and Make Up Barbie, etc. We only have a fighting chance when we recognize which Barbie we're dealing with and act accordingly.

None of that valuable experience helps in this situation. There is no Barbie for this. You will see your wife, perhaps for the first time, as the naked, vulnerable soul that she really is, and your only purpose in life from that point on is to protect her.

I'm serious. When you actually see how fragile this woman really is, you are born again. You become a new being with a single purpose. You are part warrior, part defender, part comforter, part student, part nurse, **but** fully focused on one thing: her.

And keep in mind that this new being you have become is **disposable**. You were designed to survive wounds and stress you never imagined you could withstand. You don't have armor, but you now have the ability to shed your skin and keep going. Rest for her is recouping strength and healing. Rest for you is optional.

You have no idea how much strength is inside you. Take my word for it, when you need it, it will be there.

Build a wall around her. Filter who gets in, how long they stay and what they say. Don't allow opinion, speculation or ignorance to weaken her. I don't care how well-intentioned someone is, I don't want my wife wasting energy listening to miracle cures, trendy diets or local shamans. There is a door to your house. Feel free to use it at this time. Lock it when they leave.

Keep everyone informed with the least amount of energy used by you. Sorry, individual phone calls are out of the question, there are just too many people to update. I use an email list, one email that sends the same message to everyone. If someone doesn't have email, then so be it. Ask someone on the list to keep that person informed; your energy needs to be focused on one, not many.

Her care is not an example of democracy in action. Listen carefully and then decide. When it's their turn, they will understand. Or not.

Manage the meds. She honestly doesn't remember that she took her pills two hours ago. All she knows is that it hurts.

As much as it may pain others, only you understand her most intimate communications. **The brave face she puts up for friends and family is just a**

mask, and only you can see through it. Don't ignore what you see. Get her to sanctuary, even if she protests. Sometimes she buys into her own bullshit and denies to herself how much it hurts. Take the beating later, but get her the hell out of there now. She will only suffer more the longer she stays. And hurting someone else's feelings in the process of escape is collateral damage, acceptable loss. Don't try to save everyone, just her.

Your tears are worthless. They don't solve anything; they only undermine the strength and trust your spouse sees in you. If you have to (and you will), do it on your own time and in your own space.

You don't need to be strong in *every* moment, just **this** moment.

The picture at the top of this chapter is my wedding ring.

Can You Hear Me Now?

January 17, 2011

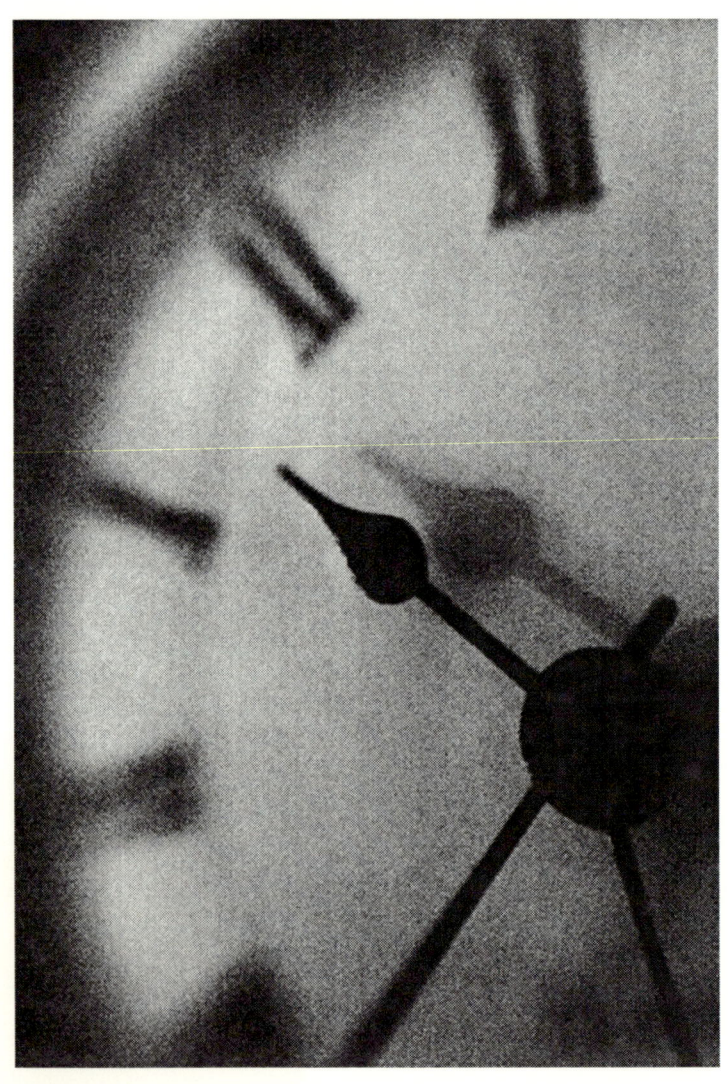

BOB MARCOTTE

Hindsight is a beautiful thing.

Over the course of years, my wife and I have learned to communicate on multiple channels. Our radio frequencies are tuned for selective communication. I use one channel to make her laugh. If that channel is being blocked because she is in pain (or in only the rarest of times, when she is mad at me) I switch to a different channel. And we go through this switching and blocking game until I get a clear signal. We seldom get our signals crossed.

It is an eloquent system of communication and it's exclusive to us. I cannot teach anyone else how to receive her messages loud and clear, in perfect context to her meaning. No, I've earned that and it's mine.

But one night, she was broadcasting on a channel she rarely uses and it concerned me greatly.

She was broadcasting on her '*I am in denial*' channel.

THE MESSAGE

The evening actually started out very pleasantly. We were celebrating the news that we had an appointment at Stanford that wasn't four months away. We were all concerned that we would have to live in limbo while waiting to be squeezed into the Stanford Cancer Center's calendar. Even when pain is "managed", limbo is still an unsettling place to live.

Conversation turned to the basic logistic questions. How are we going to get there? When would we have to leave? And then I broached the question that would trigger the conflict. It surprised me at how this question led to so much miscommunication and pure anger.

"Maybe we should stay the night so it's easier on you?"

THE MEANING

"No." (This is a blocking signal. I change frequency).

"Seriously? This is going to be tough on me, I can't imagine how you're going to feel. Let's get a room and drive back the day after".

"No. I'll be fine." (Initially I consider this as a blocking signal).

"Hey, I really don't want you to have to tough this out. You're a tough cookie but you don't need to endure all this."

"No, I'll be fine." (This is not blocking, this is now full denial. I have no idea at this time what is motivating her to think like this, to actually **believe** this, but I have to continue trying to get through).

"Carole, you don't need to suffer to get this done."

"No. I'll be fine." (This was spoken as barely a whisper, but it was the equivalent of a 911 call for me).

THE CONTEXT

What you probably don't know about Carole is her IQ. It's high. It's scary high, full 20-30 points higher than mine. (OK, maybe my IQ is not the best measuring stick available out of the whole human race, but trust me on this one, hers is high.)

Often, people with great intellects traverse the world through their intellect at the cost of artistic expression or even human compassion. (Imagine a great doctor with a lousy bedside manner). Some people with great humanity traverse the world through their greatest gift and forgo the intellectual expressions that others live by. Carole has the very rare gift of traversing the world any damn way she wants, intellectually, artistically, or spiritually.

But in those times when she is hurt or exhausted she cannot maintain all three, and she becomes very intellectual, very literal. Her responses were a signal to me that the combined stress of everything was getting to her; it was compromising her ability to evaluate. In fact, she was too overwhelmed to evaluate, that's why she'd "**be fine**". It's the answer requiring the least energy and the unspoken admission that she is very, very hurt.

MY MISTAKE

I was receiving loud and clear. I had found the broadcast channel she was using. My mistake was not to drop it.

In my own defense, there have been so many times while we've been together where injecting some imagination into the discussion awoke Carole's imagination and brain-storming would progress, solutions would be found.

But there are times where communication needs to stop. This was one of them. Perhaps in my enthusiasm to help, I went too far.

In any case, it was one too many, one too many questions, one too many attempts to unscramble the signal, one too many fill-in-the-blanks-with-whatever-you-like.

And it was perceived by Mom-in-law as disrespect of her daughter. It was perceived as having no point, and only increased her daughter's suffering. It was perceived as a heartless attack by someone who didn't care and wasn't listening. She was half-right. It didn't matter about right and wrong, she stepped in to defend her daughter...and I retreated.

AFTERMATH

By the time the dust settled, I was alone in our room seething with anger. The ladies of the house (Carole and her Mom) were on the other side of the house shaking their heads at my actions, perceived as selfishness and uncaring. (Yeah, those are **exactly** the two words I never wanted used to describe me, especially while she was suffering.) Mom-in-law was particularly and uncharacteristically vocal in her opinion, but she is from Philly so it should not come as too big a surprise....

That night Mom slept in her room, Carole slept in the living room and I barely slept in our bed. By 4:20 am I was blogging, by 7:00 am I was leaving for work.

It was a long day of coffee and energy drinks, but I was met by my wife when I returned home, and we had a very positive, very sweet conversation about it all — out of earshot of others. The next morning, again out of earshot, we came up with a plan that included everybody, and the overnight stay that I was insisting on.

It's clear to me now that I pushed too hard.

It's also clear to me that our communications just cannot be interpreted by others. She had locked her soul in a castle that night out of exhaustion and fear. A full frontal attack never works on Carole, even when she's in perfect health; it had a less-than-never change of success while she was hurt. No, the better plan would have been to drop it and try to sneak in a side door later, perhaps find the key to the issue and unlock the drawbridge, lowering it slowly at a pace she could accept.

REALITY

So, is everything back to "normal"?

The long answer is that nothing is normal right now, and hasn't been for months.

Is everyone getting along? Yup, about as well as can be expected.

The longer answer is that my wife and I are special when we are together, that communication and trust earned over almost twenty years does not translate well to others around us. We've rewired each other. Only we can communicate through the silent back channels, the privileged frequencies so rich with understanding and context.

The picture at the top of this post is of a clock in our home. It's broken, and that's what time is like in limbo.

Sometimes she cries...

January 17, 2011

She is on enough pain meds to floor Mike Tyson. This is beyond suffering, this is cruelty. Between the cancer, and the meds, and the after effects, and the pain, and the poking, and the exams, and all the damn waiting, and all of the other indignities...sometimes she cries.

She cries like the little girl she is, and always has been.
Deep, deep sobs.
Alligator tears, tears far too big for the little eyes that bore them.
And sometimes she cries...because that's all she has left.

Pain, in its many forms...

January 18, 2011

I need to clarify what led to yesterday's post.

Since the pathology on Carole's tumor (removed in December) pointed toward a source in the GI tract, the oncologist ordered a colonoscopy. Soon after we achieved a balance in the meds that controlled her pain, Carole had to start the two day process of cleansing. This process has been known to weaken healthy people.

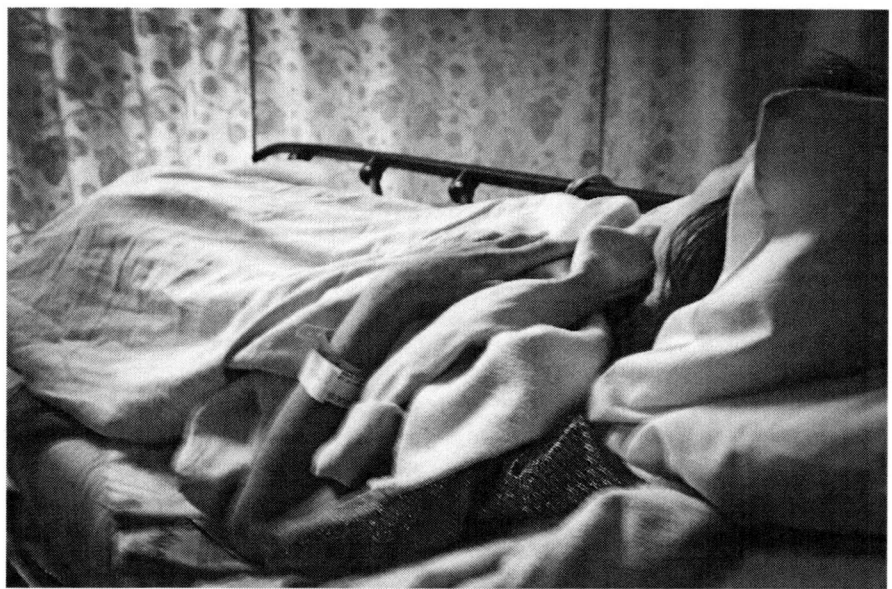

It brought Carole to her hands and knees, literally.

PAIN

Her pain meds, finally balanced and working, could not handle the additional load. She was in pain from the cancer, from the port surgery, from her guts, and she crumbled into tears. This is easily the hardest part, watching her suffer.

She endured her most brutal night so far. I know I did. I was in bed by 11:30 and up at 1:30. Two hours a night just doesn't cover it for me.

MORE PAIN

I took today off work to run errands in the morning and accompany her to the procedure this afternoon. One of the errands I had was to run to the pharmacy and pick up more pain patches.

This prescription has been cursed from the beginning. First, the pharmacist could not read the doctor's handwriting. Second, the confusion continued as the Nurse Practitioner acted as a go-between. Eventually, the confusion was lifted but now the insurance company would not pay for the increased dosage. Phone calls were made between the pharmacy and the insurance company with no resolution. The pharmacy asked me to wait while they discussed it with the doctor's office. Of course, I would have to go pick up the triplicate script (required of any narcotic) at the doctor's if they could redo it in such a way that would meet the approval of the insurance company. This had been going on since the 12th (today is the 18th) and Carole was down to her last dosage.

Sleep deprived, under pressure to keep our hospital appointment, and just generally fed up, I coughed up $165 for the pain meds my wife needed. Forget the premiums, forget the co-pay, I paid solely to relieve her pain.

MY EPIPHANY

As I waited for the script to be filled, I walked over to the cooler, past the booze, and to the energy drinks. I opened it on the way back to the waiting area. No employee questioned me as I sat, drank, and considered the predicament.

Somewhere, someone had assembled a spreadsheet that dictated how much pain my wife was allowed. Someone, after yet another good night's sleep, decided that people who needed this kind of pain relief would have to do a better job of proving it. You don't get what you don't deserve.

At that moment, I made a commitment. I either needed to adhere to the Mayan calendar and die in spectacular fashion in the next twelve months, or I had to start reading the bus schedules so I could throw myself in front of a bus and thereby control the exact time and place of my demise.

You see, all of this was to lessen the load on my over-burdened insurance company. No frivolous prescriptions or pain meds for me, no confusing dosages. Nope, I would be the best insuree they had ever insured. Think of it as 'Soylent Green' meets fiscal sobriety.

CLARITY

Our world is so upside down that this solution is as valid as any other. Watching my wife crawl on hands and knees to the sink just to stand up is cruel. Having an insurance company deny the existence of such pain is just another insult, another indignity in this whole process.

And for the record, we were called by the local hospital and asked to come in early for testing. We arrived before noon for a 1:30 pm procedure. As of 3 pm, we were still waiting for an anesthesiologist. Adding insult to injury, after the procedure the complimentary valet parking staff lost my car and Carole had to sit there while they located it. No problem guys, it's just pain.

And the additional testing we were asked to arrive early for ended up not being required.

LIVES DIM

Welcome to our reality, one seemingly designed to drain our finances, our patience, and our lives. Cancer, it seems, may not be the greatest challenge before us.

THE "N" WORD

Carole's Mom arrives again in a little over twelve hours. You seldom hear married men say this, but I need my Mother-In-Law here and now.

And yes, I said **need**.

You sometimes can win a battle alone. It often takes a completely fearless and uninformed view of the odds, but sometimes bravado can win the day. But this is war, a series of seemingly endless battles. A single heart may have the desire to fight until the end, but the reality of life is that I need help in the most supreme definition of the word 'need'. There are too many battles for the heartbeats I have. As much as I love her, I only have so many heartbeats.

I can be stubborn, and while that can be a charming trait, it is not enough to win a war.

A well-working ice maker, a dirty glass and a decent whiskey (or scotch) is certainly required, but they are not the secret weapon that solves every problem.

I need her Mom, all five feet two inches and eighty-two years of her. She has a magic that even I cannot master.

My wife listens to her.

My sleep lately has been a very deep and dreamless sleep, more a coma than rest. I waken as if I never slept, and that should have been a clue that I was burning out. The coincidence that many friends approached me recently wanting to discuss stress relief was also a big clue. I guess my urge to punch people was a signal to the sane ones that the caregiver was approaching insanity.

Graceland for the Gaseous

January 19, 2011

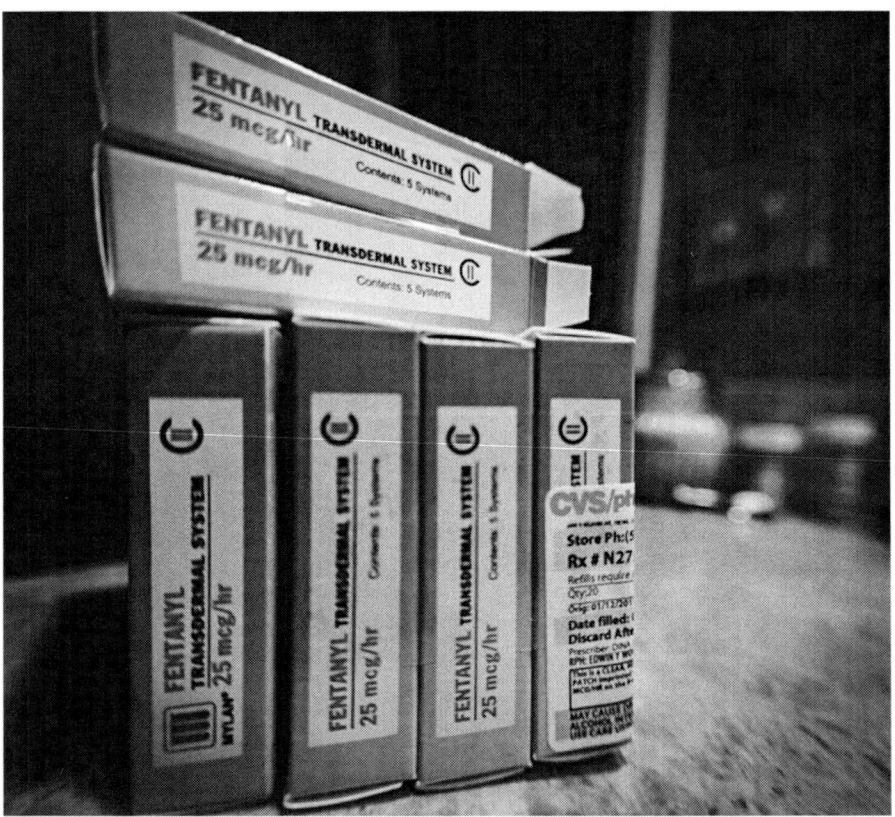

Dear Readers, I know the blog has been particularly heavy as of late, and for this I am sorry.

Today I want to share with you a lighter phenomenon that I have seen in various places during our trip through the medical establishment. Perhaps you have seen it for yourself.

While the endoscopy department was quietly humming with conversations and activities, a certain patient was escorted in. It was clear from the outset that this patient was unlike most of the patients within earshot. I will call the patient 'A.W.'.

A.W. was here for more than treatment. This was his place to get the all important attention that he must have lacked as a child. This was a place that truly understood him. In fact, this was not A.W's first time here. No this was his second, third or maybe fifth encore.

You see... **A.W. WAS HERE TO PERFORM!**

He warmed up with a few standard questions from the nurse and then it was showtime! When asked why he was getting a colonoscopy, he answered with his voice raised, his chin high **"Honey, I haven't had a colon since 1997!"**

With that, he caught the attention of everyone around him. Even the zombies in the waiting room watching Dr. Phil had to break away from their reverie. Yes, it was showtime! The curtain had risen!

"Sweetie, if you can give me a colonoscopy, I would love you forever!"

From this point on the answers came fast and furious. The nurse was almost acting as his straight man, feeding him opportunities to wow the crowd with his medical history, his command of big words, and his insistence on calling his doctor by first name.

Oh yes, this patient was a patient among patients, a star waiting to be scoped, a talent of suffering so large as to dwarf the suffering of those around him. This was a major league patient in a minor league clinic.

He was a pro.

"I will pay the insurance deductible if the nurse will put the guy in the bed next to us out for the afternoon." ~ Twittered by me at intermission!

After they gave him a bed and his examination gown, Act II began.

Oh, he was good. He played for laughs, he played for tears. I've seen good theater in my day and this was it. Well-written, well-rehearsed and delivered like Paul Lynd in the center square. Timing like a Swiss watch, and not a cue card in sight.

When asked a leading question by the attention deficit nurse, he lowered his voice (but not enough so the people in the parking garage would miss a word) and told about how he remembered his first colonoscopy.

If there was any justice in the world, the lights would have dimmed, the strings come in quietly and he would have sung his Broadway hit, the "***Ballad of the Missing Bowels***". Tears would have poured from the box seats to the cheap seats and pooled at his feet. Yes, this was an artist in his realm, at the very top of his game. Somewhere in the world they give awards for performances like these. I wished he was there.

THE BIG FINISH

And then, with a lightning transition, the lights would have come up, and he would have gone for the big ending. Top hat, white tails, a walking cane and dancing sigmoids, all with feathery fans.

A kick line! Yes, a kick line with him in the center, wrapped in a boa the same length as his missing bowels! (Visual aids are always helpful).

EXIT STAGE LEFT

When it was his turn, they rolled him stage left and he waved, and he literally thanked every nurse by name. The feeling among the audience was applause, applause and more applause.

Or not.

I believe the audience was feeling relief more than anything else. This guy robbed a lot of people of energy, and his descriptions of medical procedures, while technically accurate and dramatically delivered, were scaring people hoping to avoid such things.

A.W. (Attention Whore) had raised many of the fears that so many people in that room there were trying to control. He had reminded people of thoughts they were trying so hard to suppress.

I desperately wanted to say "Goodbye, Asshole" but I was afraid that too would have been treated as a song cue, just another in a long line of numbers about his medical history.

The picture at the top of this post is the stuff that allows us to keep what sense of humor we have left.

You mean, besides the cancer?

January 21, 2011

As a doctor walks through a hospital, he is master of all he surveys. He's the Lion, and everyone in the pride defers to him. The nurses, the technicians, hospital staff and pharmacists, all well educated themselves, await his arrival, follow his 'orders'.

And the hospital itself is spread over acres. Most hospitals offer complimentary valet parking, because it's cheaper than sending out search parties for patients who have lost their cars.

The complex is the size of a man-made mountain, and a river runs through it. A river of humanity; pushed by the same flow, the flow of survival, of discomfort, of anxiety. Every time the doors open, more people are pushed through. The river runs and never stops.

And at every significant turn through this jungle, you meet another person foreign to you. They are trained to ask questions, to learn your purpose for being here and push you down yet another tributary, to another department, to another interrogator.

Of course, they need to ask questions but there is one that is the most painful to hear – *"Are there any significant health issues we need to be aware of?"*

We used to be confused and hurt by this, but now we have a stock answer designed as much to shock the interrogator as inform them.

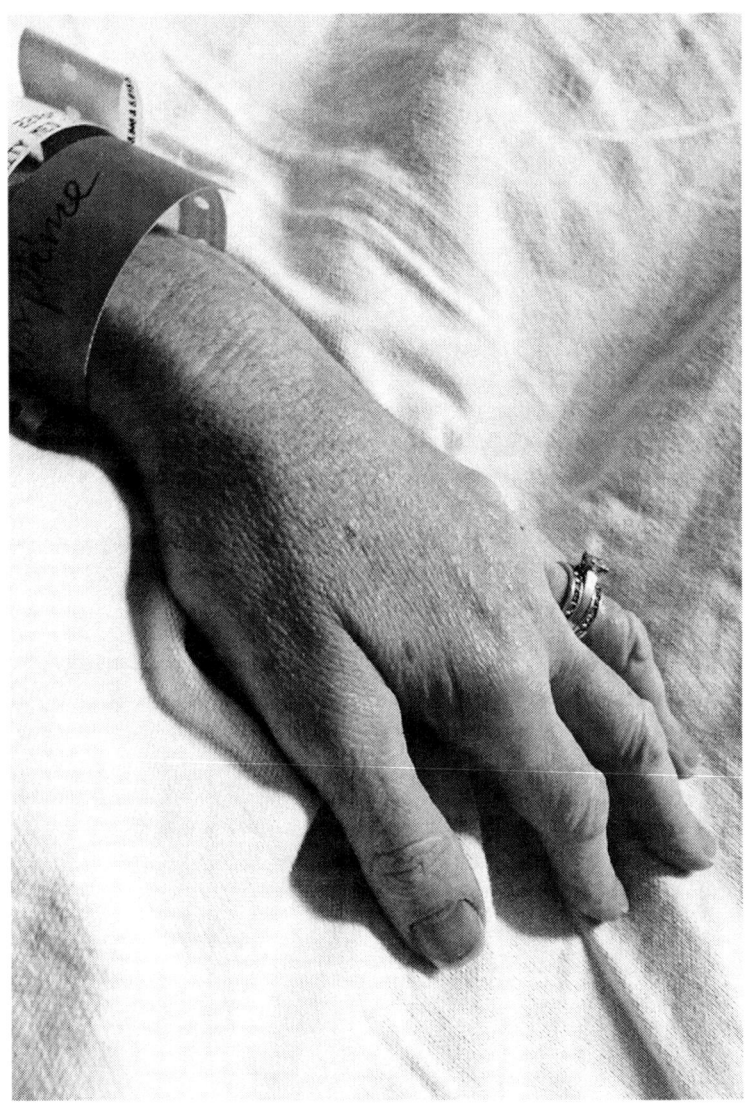

"You mean, besides the cancer?"

FRAGILE, HANDLE WITH CARE

Every day, delicate and precious items are shipped throughout the world; anything from sensitive computer gear, glass, or art, to human organs. These shipments are labeled as "Fragile". That typically informs the people responsible for shipping to treat this box differently, sometimes even gingerly.

As we drift through the medical system, why can't there be a label, a badge, a bracelet that says "Fragile, Handle With Care", a way to alert the caregivers that this patient is not here for the mundane head cold or sprained ankle, but that this patient is at a point in her physical health where her emotional strength is waning.

Listen, we realize that the world does not revolve around our care, but the result of being asked this question over and over again is a loss of identity, a sense of isolation, and a sense of being very, very small in this man-made jungle, inside the man-made mountain, in the middle of acres of parking, at the mercy of Lions.

I am Carole's guide. I will not allow indignities like these to turn into the crushing weight that some people must feel as they drift through a terrain like this alone. Their sense of self must be compressed so small that they feel insignificant, unwanted, a pest like ants on the jungle floor, or worse.

Extinct.

Pre-school

January 22, 2011

Well, I have a birthday coming up. It's not a "milestone" birthday, I just crossed one of those last year. Honestly, the significance of my birth seems far more important to a select group than it does me.

It's not that I didn't give it a moment of retrospect; I have. I have tried to live a life filled with more saving graces than damning accusations, but as I grow older I admit to losing my patience a little more, especially at the self-entitled who live off of someone else's money and achievement. I guess it's a pet peeve brought on by the double whammy of a crashed economy and a vanquished retirement fund.

This precipice I now find myself on does provide a longer view of past and present though. I see further and more calmly, in both directions, with more clarity. I admit that the future still scares me, as it did when I was younger, but now it's perhaps a little scarier, since it's more real.

As a younger man, all I wanted to do is something, *anything* to "*make a difference*". How did I do? As my friends in accounting would say, let's look at the numbers:

65 pounds overweight.

$2,500 saved for retirement.

I do know that there are *zero* trophies on my shelf, no "I Love Me" wall of degrees and diplomas, no "Thank You" cards from presidents and prime ministers.

Over a million notes played, some of them even played well. (I do regret not having taken music seriously when I was younger, not even for a single day.)

And an *unknown* number of differences made.

But perhaps the first full fifty years of my life can be summed up in one elegant, all-encompassing phrase:

Pre-school.

The day Carole and I heard the words "cancer" and "positive" in the same sentence from the doctor now stands as Milestone Day. Worthy of being remembered year after year, more so than the day a different doctor slapped my ass to make me take my first breath.

The first fifty years were really just spent searching for "meaning" and chasing diversions. Now, I can truly say that life has a purpose, not one that I ever would have expected or volunteered for, but a purpose made of immoveable concrete. This purpose will withstand earthquakes, fires, floods, and any other damn thing that gets thrown our way.

It's inside this concrete purpose that I hide her. Nothing from the outside will hurt her while she is this weak, nothing from the inside will threaten her.

On Tuesday, my wife has a hair appointment and will have her beautiful hair cut short. She wants to do it on her terms and not watch it fall out from cancer or chemo.

During that same appointment I am having what little of my hair is left shaved off. She is free to decide if I will keep the beard or lose everything. I don't care what the world sees, I only care that she sees someone as committed as she is, follicle-ly or otherwise, to her comfort and survival.

It's my intent to only grow back my hair when she grows hers. We'll simply spend less on shampoo and more on shaving cream and razors.

And on the day after that, we're heading to Stanford for further examination, discussion and opinion. (The irony is not lost on me that we will be passing ORACLE on the way. Aren't we doing exactly what kings and princes did in ancient times, seeking answers?)

I mention all this to make a point. I could never have taken this on ten years ago, or twenty. The effort required for this purpose is not about youth as much as it is about wisdom, calm, and a toughness earned by the world continuing to beat my ass from day one.

Call it God, call it coincidence or karma, I don't care. It's all Pre-School. Real-School starts in a few weeks. The tests are brutal (more on her than me) but I am just old enough now to return that brutality with compassion, fidelity, and an equal brutality if required.

I sincerely don't care if I have to retire to the streets and fight dogs for scraps, I now have my purpose.

And soon, I will have a healthy wife and a degree from the only school that matters — life.

Droppin' Dimes

January 24, 2011

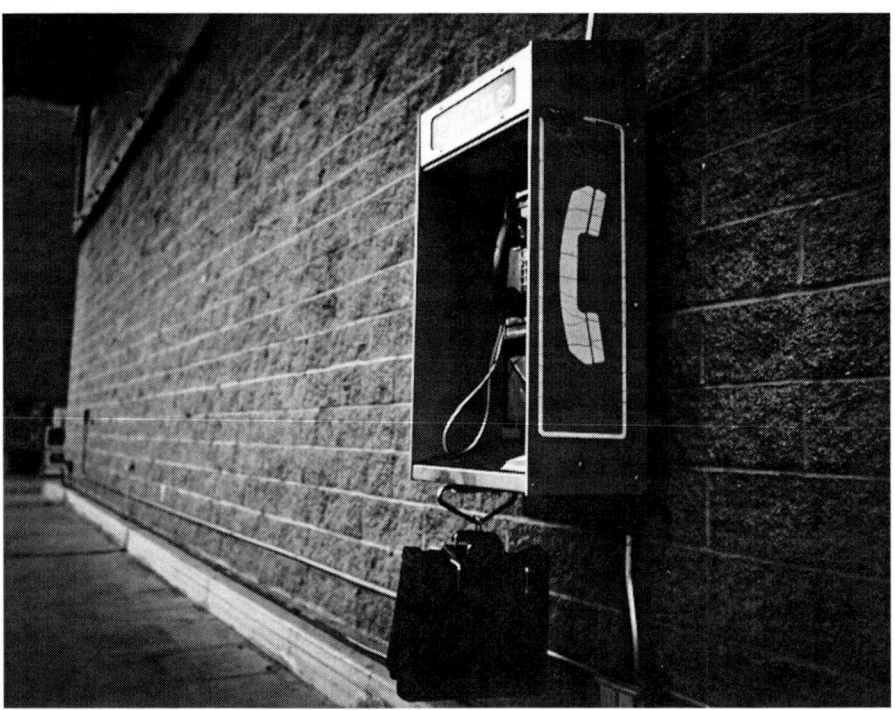

It's 3:30 AM and I am holding my wife's hand as she endures yet another wave of pain. It's worse at night for some reason. The pain meds that "manage" the pain seem to go to sleep when it gets dark, unlike my wife, and often unlike me.

Most people who know me realize that while I don't have a hard time believing in God, I don't always believe in all the people running around in pointy hats who organize "organized" religion.

Religious affiliations aside, at times like these, people sometimes pray. They pray for rest, for relief from pain, for mercy or some sense of peace. It's at a time like this that I also might "drop a dime" on Jesus. "Droppin' a dime on Jesus" is a phrase heard often in old blues tunes. It means to say a prayer, a specific prayer asking for something that seems impossible without God's intervention, like relieving punishing pain in a loved one.

(Note to younger readers: there used to be these little boxes called "phone booths" all over the place where you could make a call from a "pay phone", a dime for three minutes. I realize that some of you think of this as archaic technology, and rightly so. The average lifespan of a new technology is now down to eighteen months; however, people used these phone booths, especially when they were too poor to own their own phone. People would go down to the corner and make a call at all hours of the night; typically as they watched dinosaurs roam the earth. OK, that last part isn't true but I figured I'd just verbalize what some of you youngsters were already thinking.)

Getting back on topic, in a stressful time where a feeling of helplessness permeates all thought, prayer, at least for some people, becomes an option.

But I often wonder if my calls are even getting through.

Faith without question to me is not faith at all. Faith in that case becomes just a set of instructions, a computer program, like following a GPS turn by turn. In fact, I'm sure there are people who have more faith in their GPS than in God. And some days I understand why.

On more than one occasion recently, I have pondered just what the hell is going on. What purpose is all this pain serving? What purpose does any pain serve, except to teach us that the oven is hot, or running with scissors can lead to some serious discomfort?

It's at times like last night, when my prayers and support seem to make no difference to my spouse, when the doubt and questioning begins. I'm not a robot. I find it impossible to watch my wife suffer and not feel for her. I want it fixed. I question why it's happening. I plead with the "Big Guy" asking for relief, for the meds to kick in quickly, for a miracle if we somehow qualify for that level of consideration (and just what do we have to do to get to that level of consideration?). It's strange to me that the Bible is filled with miracles far greater than what I'm asking for, but nothing happens here. I am not asking to walk on water or raise the dead, just give this innocent woman a single, quiet night's sleep.

But the next morning, the sunrise and too much coffee often brings a different perspective. To see how friends and family have galvanized to support us and protect us is a small miracle. To see the sincere compassion poured out over us on a daily basis is a miracle. The level of this compassion we have been given is far greater than either of us knew existed in our world.

A piece of that compassion that we hear a lot is that people are praying for us. That's a good thing, since I often find myself too tied up in this moment's challenge to ask for help on a regular basis. But the prayers of others **are** having an effect in our lives.

That's when I question what it is *I* am praying for.

Perhaps what I am asking for is not "mercy", but "control".

It's at times like these that I remember the prayer my mother taught me as a child, the one that says **"thy will be done on earth, as it is in heaven"**. I don't wear a pointy hat in an organized religion, but the implication of those words to me is that my wife's pain is not God's will. In fact, it implies that not much of what happens on earth these days is God's will.

I don't have a degree in theology, but even I know the textbook answer to your question. Why is God's will not being done? Because of Adam, because of human free will, because humans think they can conceive and control everything they lay eyes on. Don't get me wrong, the human spirit can be a wonderful thing, but human spirit without conceit is hard to find. You just don't cure a disease without taking a bow, you know? And how do you justify taking ALL the credit when the Creator is watching?

In this case, as much as I still believe in the "Big Guy", I confess that I would be the first to stand and applaud the person who finds the cure for my wife's disease. I would organize the parades, I would throw the ticker tape and hand her the award she so richly deserves.

Desperate people make desperate deals. At those times when all I can do is squeeze her hand, I would do anything to find her cure and ease her pain, whether it came from Adam's Creator, or Adam's Offspring. The pointy hats need not intrude; this theology is born of a pain I can not relieve or control. Yes, I said control, because my wife's comfort means that much to me.

Yup, I am a person whose faith is being more seriously tested than in any other time in my life. This is a believer hanging on to belief in time of great doubt. I am a human, feeling what it means to be fully human, fully helpless, fully at the mercy of someone or something that can make a difference if I somehow make my plea heard.

This is going to be a tough week of doctor appointments, capped off by a visit to Stanford. For the record, I will accept help from any corner at any time, and I'll be swinging by the bank tomorrow. My guess is that even with Stanford's help, I'll be needing lots of dimes.

Laps

January 25, 2011

When I was a kid, I used to imagine that the track surrounding the high school football field was a year, and that every corner of the track was a transition.

That far corner, shaded by trees, was always the dark corner. It was the last corner to get sun, and the snow remained there longer than anyplace else on the field. That corner was the chill of a New England November. That corner also held the dark winter of December and the even darker cold of January. As you finally rounded that far corner, you turned into February, and the optimism that baseball spring training brought. Soon, the weather would warm, that last snow would melt and I could play outside, and of course, follow the Red Sox for another heartbreaking season.

In 2010, I had three jobs at one point to offset my wife's forced unemployment. One of those three jobs I actually loved. I was a free-lance photographer for the Fresno Bee Custom Publications department. I was sent all over the Central Valley to get shots of all kinds of events that make up the life of this valley. One of those assignments was to a small, pretty town called Exeter, to shoot the American Cancer Society 'Relay for Life'. People who were survivors, or family members, friends and even neighbors committed to walk the track around the high school football field for 24 hours, to raise money to fight cancer. Initially, I wondered just how much money could be raised by a small town to fight cancer, and if this event would make any difference to anybody. That thought fell out of my head as I drove down there. A gig was a gig and I needed the money.

Many things caught my eye that day. It was an easy gig to shoot as these things went. The story was right there before me everywhere I turned. My favorite reporter, David, was with me, and he asked me to get certain shots as his ideas started flowing. I not only like David, I trust him. He and I see the world in much the same way, except he uses words and I used only pictures then. And every picture was dripping with meaning. There was laughter and much joy to be sure, but it was countered by a solemn purpose. These people all knew something that I didn't. They didn't know each other's names at times, but the looks they exchanged were spiritual connections. In fact, at some points I felt a little uncomfortable intruding on their intimacy.

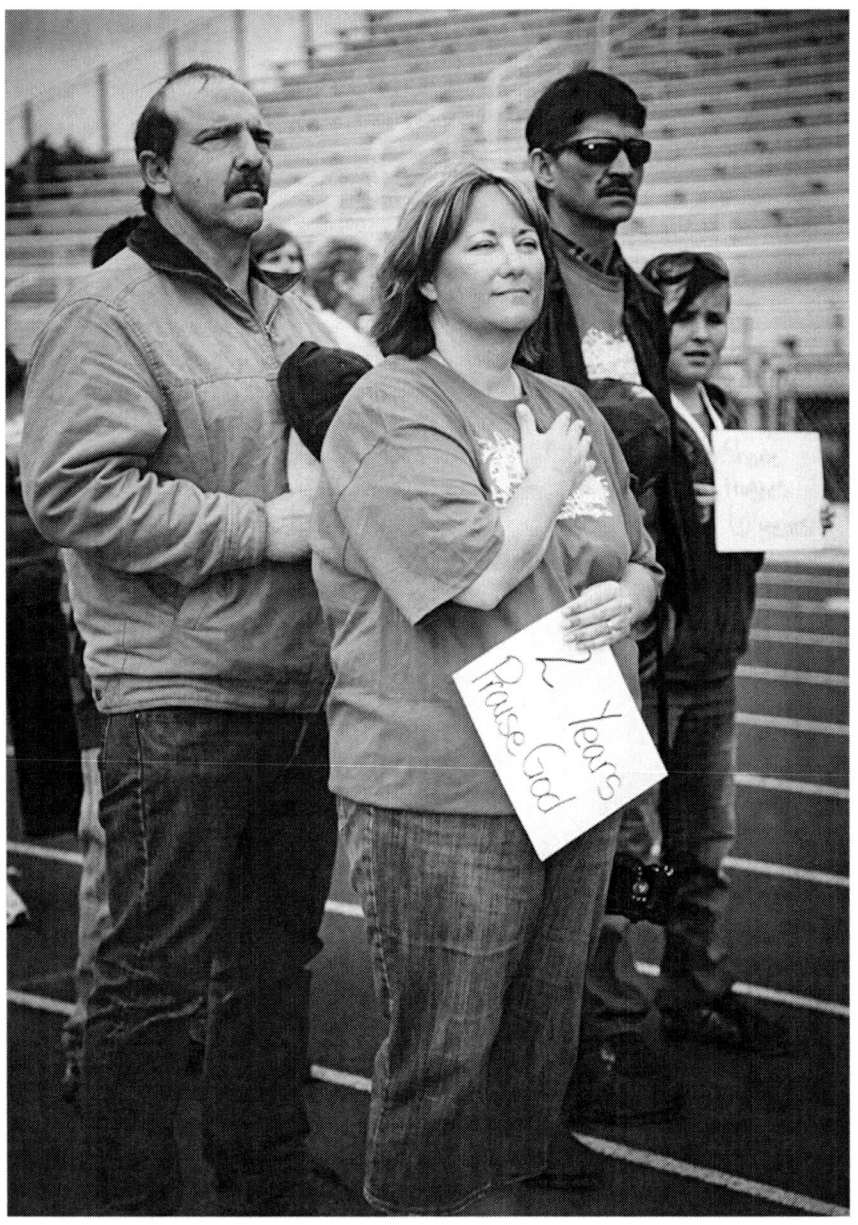
Little did I know I was walking amid my future family.

PURPLE IS A ROYAL COLOR

Survivors were honored by wearing a purple shirt. I was surprised and pleased at how much purple surrounded me. Survivors were encouraged to carry signs stating how long they'd been cancer-free. They celebrated every moment they were "clean", they mourned the people who were here just a year ago, and supported those who were in the midst of their battle, some for the second or even third time.

Family and friends were encouraged to create custom luminaria, white bags weighed down by sand with a candle inside. These bags were decorated with the names of someone dearly missed, or of someone who dearly needed the support that only such medically trivial creations can give. David and I were really not there that long, just a few hours, but by the time we were leaving, the bags, placed by volunteers, were stretching halfway around the track. That night, the candles would be lit, and friends and family would walk the high school track illuminated by hopes and prayers. This was no longer a high school track, it was becoming hallowed ground. A place where horrible pasts, difficult presents and uncertain futures met shaken faith, hope beyond all hope and unconditional love. Medically trivial, spiritually enormous.

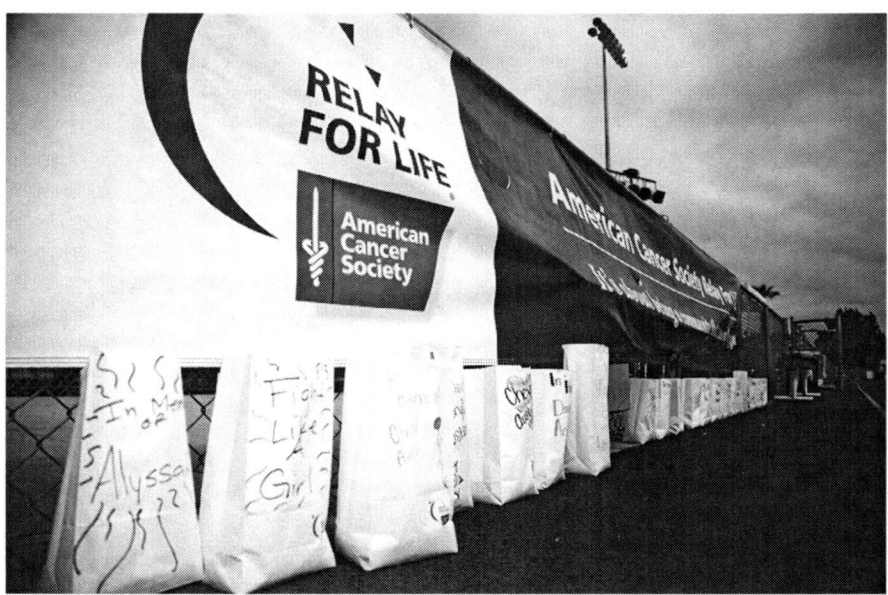

Even in my ignorance, I was touched by just how many of these bags were on the track, and how many more were waiting to be placed. I took pictures (that I later decided not to submit to the editor) of an eight year old girl coloring a white bag asking God to save her father who was sitting next to her. He wore the shirt of a survivor, but he was recently informed that the cancer had returned. Clean for a decade, but now thrown back into the fight for his life. And the little girl continued to draw and color, with the concentration that only a little girl can put into a creation pleading for her Daddy's life. No, I put my camera down after a few frames. This intimate moment did not need to be seen. The story could be told with other less powerful and far less intimate images. I still have the images; they're still too emotionally raw to post.

I CANNOT COLOR OR DRAW

It came to me that these posts are really all I have. These are my pleadings, wrapped around a track of what seems like time frozen, an effort of trivial medical value. Unlike the survivors I photographed, Carole and I have no experience with what is around the next corner. We can't 'see' the turns, we don't know what lies ahead. All we know is that we're walking as far as we have to, and we're walking together. Our appointment to hear the results from Stanford is set for February 2nd. I hope that corner of the track still has its February optimism, that the weather will warm and life become a little easier, day by day. But somehow, I believe that life will become tougher before it becomes easier. You see, we don't know where we are on the track.

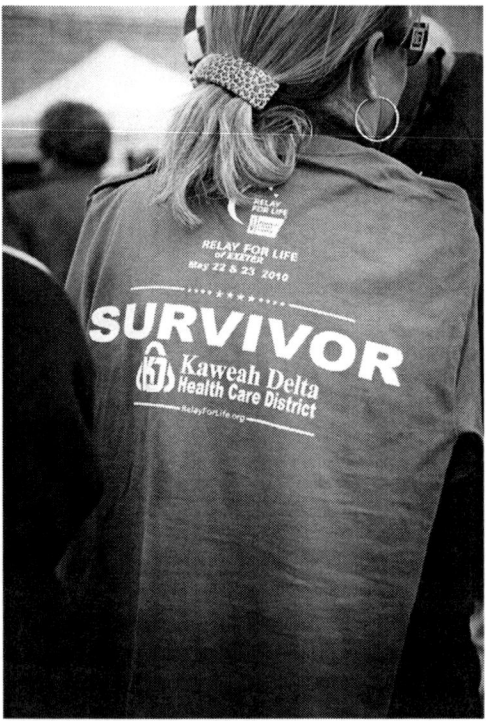

The picture above is a shirt I very much look forward to buying for my wife. My wife looks really good in purple.

A Fog, Only Less

January 29, 2011

Six days ago, Carole's sister arrived from the East Coast. Her flights were all on time until she got to San Francisco. Her flight could not leave S.F. because the fog in Fresno was so thick they could not land. This early morning, I dropped Sis off at the same Fresno airport in the same fog, just a bit less. Her flight should be able to get out on time. While driving home, it occurred to me that the fog and this family have something in common. After an exciting, and at times dramatic week, we were still in a fog as far as Carole's condition and care is concerned. But the fog is lifting.

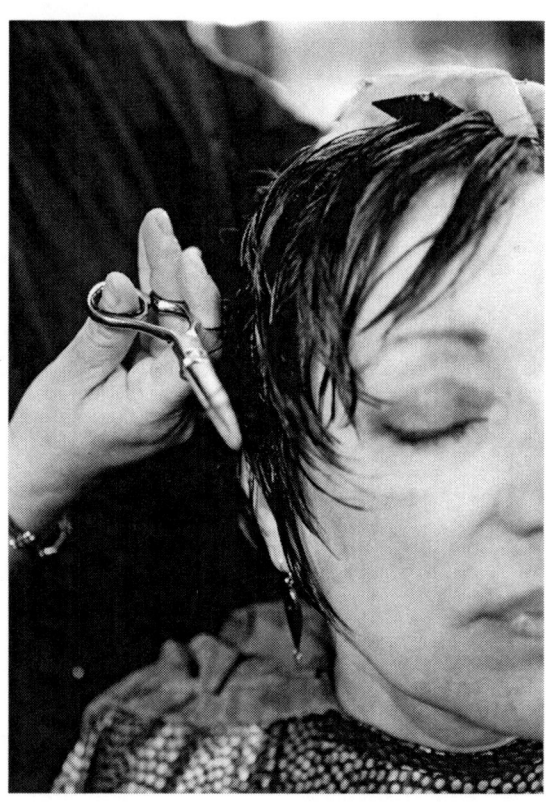

The week really started on Tuesday. It was my fifty-first birthday, we were preparing for a trip to Stanford the next day, but, more importantly, in anticipation of having to endure six months of chemo, it was the day Carole decided to cut her hair.

Mom and Sis made sure that this hair appointment would be as uplifting and joyous as possible. Food was prepared, wine was chilled and the party started the minute we arrived. Clients of the salon were invited to share in the goodies and the event. Soon everyone knew about "the haircut" and support poured out from friends and strangers. Buoyed by liquid courage, Carole sat in the chair and watched as her hair fell to the floor.

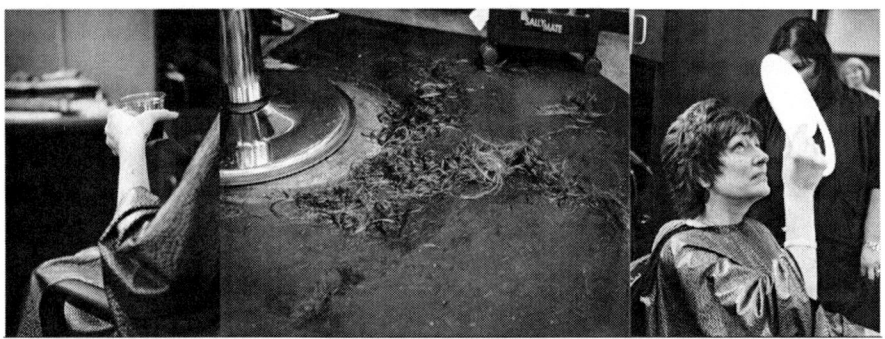

Compliments flew her way as her hair was shaped, but the few times we could make uninterrupted eye contact I could see her reservation, not so much about the hair but about the future.

THE LONGEST DAY

Thanks to two wonderful friends who let us borrow their Lincoln Navigator (technically an SUV but more like a living room on wheels), we were able to get Carole, her Mom, her Sis and me to Stanford. It was like we had a private ambulance. Carole laid down in the back row and slept when she could, and the rest of us either took care of her, drove, or helped navigate.

We arrived with the expectation that the slides (tissue samples from Carole's three surgeries) had been sent ahead of us for evaluation. We were immediately disappointed with the news that Stanford had no record of them. We had, however, hand carried a DVD of images from Carole's most recent CT and PET scans. Those images were evaluated while we waited and then we met the woman who would change everything.

Our doctor is a diminutive Asian woman, but she speaks with great authority. As best as I can recall, these were the words she used to change everything:

"Far be it from me to tell another doctor how to practice medicine, but your doctors are wrong."

At this point, had an earthquake hit Palo Alto, I would not have noticed. Everything I read, everything I was led to believe vanished when I finally exhaled.

She went on to explain that the tumor is not of G.I. origin and that chemo would have no effect on this cancer. Furthermore, radiation is the treatment course, and you need to start very soon. The only question in her mind was whether any surgeon at Stanford would consider removing what parts of the tumor they thought they could remove before radiation, or just go straight to the radiation. She said this would be a difficult and tricky surgery since the tumor was invading the coccyx, sacrum, and the nerves below (she referred to the nerves as the "horse tail"), but successful surgery is what the surgeons at Stanford were known for. Coincidentally, the tumor board met weekly on Wednesdays, and she wanted to present this case to them – today.

(It's at about this time that I wished the chair I was sitting in had seat belts and an airbag!)

We arrived at Stanford at about 10 am. We saw the doctor at about noon, and then again at about 5:30 pm, after the board meeting. She informed us that the surgeons declined the case but only because they were G.I. surgeons and that this was an OB/GYN case. (It's at this point that I realized the misdiagnosis from Fresno had referred us to the wrong department at Stanford.)

In our previous meeting, she asked why the doctors treating Carole allowed her to be in so much pain. Even though she could not give us definitive treatment answers at this point, she could lessen Carole's pain. In three mighty signatures, she prescribed an increase in Carole's pain medication (Fentanyl), some 'pops' (basically Fentanyl on a stick, short acting pain relief for "break-through" pain) and the most amazing steroid. This steroid is used to reduce swelling, especially on cancer patients. It shrinks the tumor, and thereby relieves pain.

By about 7 pm I walked out of the pharmacy (conveniently located in the lobby) with a **HUGE** bag of pain meds for Carole. The bag could have easily fit two Whoppers, two large fries and still had room for dessert. Sis had retrieved the car from valet and had loaded the family in. When she saw me coming towards the car with such a large bag she is reported to have said, "Here comes the Candy Man".

THE MONTEREY MIRACLE

Our original plan was to go to Stanford and then down to Monterey, to show Mom and Sis one of our favorite places in all of California. Think of it as a vacation from cancer. After taking the steroid pill and trying her 'pop', Carole laid down in the back of the van and slept as we drove to Monterey. Everyone, including myself, was exhausted from all the driving, the waiting and the news of the day.

I must have slept like a rock that night, since I didn't recall Carole tossing and turning, or moaning in pain, as was now common these last four months. As I opened my eyes the next morning I saw Carole standing with a look of surprise on her face. She summed it up this way:

"It's smaller. I slept all night and the tumor is smaller, I can feel it!"

In my own defense, I took this incredible news lying down, because we had received so much incredible news in the last twenty-four hours that I think I would have fallen.

And, as if Stanford wasn't impressive enough, BOTH our cell phones were filled with messages from Stanford trying to book appointments for Friday (tomorrow) in Radiation Oncology and OB/GYN oncology. It was 8:15 am.

A FOG, ONLY LESS

In the end, we scheduled appointments for Stanford for Monday. They were even kind enough to book us starting at 1 pm, because they knew we were driving in from Fresno.

Yesterday, I got to the bottom of the "slides" drama, and even have a copy of the pathology report. This information is (supposed to be) at Stanford now, but I'll carry a copy just in case.

Carole's pain right now is well-managed. She can move, she can sleep, she has life back in hers eyes, she is optimistic. Whether you chalk this up to God or medical competency, it's still a miraculous change, and it put me on my knees in thanks. We're still waiting to formulate the plan of attack, but it's so much easier without the suffering. We WILL beat cancer if we keep getting help like this from friends, family and medical science.

And that diminutive Asian woman who was a stranger to us last week is now my hero. All I ever asked for was for someone, something to relieve my wife's pain. It's no longer a coincidence to me that some doctors and angels dress in white. They are one and the same.

And the hair? It will grow back, in the future; the future that I was so unsure about last week, the future that I am starting to believe in more and more today.

All I can do is say thank you.

I make this look good

January 30, 2011

Finally, I found the time to finish the haircut that started Tuesday, the day when Carole cut her hair. You can say that the cue ball is polished, the dome is chromed, or that my forehead now ends at my ass cheeks...

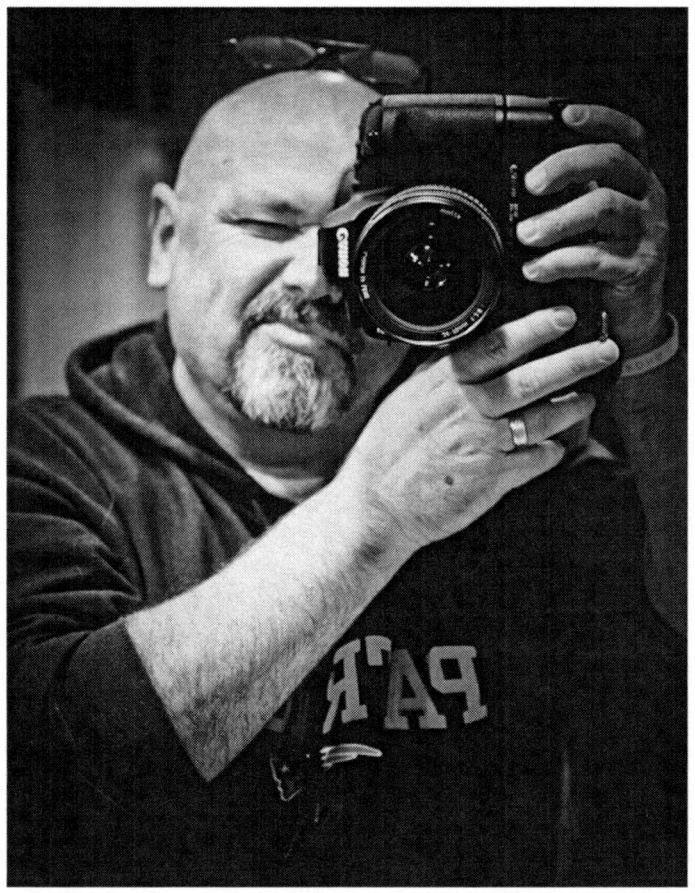

...as long as you remember why I did it.

The Beach

January 31, 2011

The cliff was steep but manageable. I carried her in my arms, but she was weightless.

My bare feet eventually touched the sand, that transition between life and afterlife. Here the sand was part dry, part wet, partly here and partly there.

I held her in the water as the gentle waves rose and fell. I did not let the water cover her face. She was gone, but I still would not let her drown.

As the water washed over her, her eyes opened and she gave me her most loving, content smile. It was the best smile of all our time together.

Her blue eyes danced against the color of the water, and then she was free. Like a mammal released from captivity, she gracefully rolled from my arms. She swam and danced and dove and played in the water, her joy uncontainable. Like an otter, she twisted and rolled and floated on her back. With one last wordless look my way, she dove beneath the waves and was truly gone. I knew that was our good bye.

I stared at the water a little longer, hoping for some sign that she was all right, but I knew that she was, and that she would not show herself again.

The waves that welcomed her were now pushing back against me. "Go back," they seemed to say. "You cannot swim, it is not your time."

And slowly, reluctantly I turned for shore, feeling as if I would miss her if I completely turned my back to the waves. It's at that time I noticed that the beach was long, and that it was filled with people like me, people freeing loved ones from pain.

And as I took a slow deep breath, I finally allowed myself to believe she was really gone.

Above me I noticed people on the top of the cliff, not really looking at me as much as looking past me. They were all very aware of what I had just done, but in their denial they could not look directly at me. They were faceless, but I knew them all. I wanted to shake them, to warn them that they may someday take my place in the waves, but their denial was too strong, it drowned out my caring, my alarm.

I stood on the dry sand, the place that was fully mine. For one last time I took a long look at the water, the ever-moving waves. So much saltwater, and none of it from tears. It was the place of lasting joy and vanquished pain. It was the place of wholeness, and happiness, and fulfillment.

And it was not mine; it was not my time; the waves told me so. Mine was the destiny of more pain, more searching, more emptiness, but this time with no purpose or identity. I was born to comfort her, care for her, but now she didn't need me. She was perfectly at peace, and I was perfectly destroyed.

As I climbed the cliffs, my legs began to hurt. It was just small preview of what lies ahead.

And then I heard an alarm. My alarm?

I open one eye and there it stands, beeping and flashing, informing me that I need to get up, that today we drive to Stanford and meet with the doctors who will form a plan of attack to make her life whole again.

No, not all dreams come true, especially this one.

No, today is the first real step we take to keeping our dreams intact, the dreams we both share.

Time to get up.

A Question of God

January 31, 2011

Wouldn't it be wonderful if once in your life you could hit the "pause" button, stop life and ask one deeply sincere, honest question of God?

I'm afraid I would have used up my one question many times over when it comes to my wife.

I would have asked, "Is she the one, my life partner?" The answer was yes, with apologies to all those who were hurt by it, especially my son.

In 2003 and 2006, I would have asked, "Will she survive?" In both cases, the answer was yes.

Now, in 2011, my question is different. The question now is, "What is it?"

You see, I have held back some information. The latest pathology of the specimen recovered in December of 2010 is inconclusive, as are the pathologies from 2003 and 2006. Just to be clear, the findings are not only about what kind of cancer Carole has, but whether or not it's even cancer.

THE PATHOLOGY

There is no question that Carole has a tumor (just another word for growth or mass) at the base of her spine near the tail bone (coccyx). This tumor involves the sacrum and the cauda equina. The tumor also involves the bones of her pelvis. It is a slow-growing mass that is leaning into nerves and surrounding bones, arteries and organs (her right kidney). Nowhere in any report is the word "malignancy" used, and that is the professional word for cancer.

There is discussion and (professional) disagreement among the Stanford docs about what the tumor is and where it comes from. From my limited understanding, if this were cancer, it would know if it's a copy or the original (primary). The specimens don't know that. Also, if this were cancer, it would respond to testing and tell us if it were an ovarian cancer, or a cancer from the G.I. tract. In other words, it would tell us by its genetic makeup what it is, and therefore how to kill it. Some cancers you kill with chemo, some with radiation.

In Carole's case, every test is indefinite. Not only does that cloud the question of how to treat it, it also clouds **who** treats it. The G.I. doc says it's ovarian, and therefore the responsibility of OB/GYN. (Again, this is her opinion; there is no science to support this).

The OB/GYN surgeon says that anytime the G.I. docs are confused, they blame it on the ovaries.

And Stanford is so professional; they can have discussions like this with patients and not undermine the other doctors. It's clear that these healers only care about the patient, not about bragging rights.

THE PLAN

So, in the best interest of the patient, this burden has fallen to the Radiology Oncology docs. Why? Because any way you look at it, this thing has to be stopped and shrunk to provide pain relief and give surgeons options about removing it.

Again, the professionalism of Stanford shines through. When asked what the typical course of treatment is for this condition, the answer we got from the doctor was "I don't know; we've never seen this before".

Yup, a medical anomaly. We're treading on new medical ground, as least as far as Stanford Pathology; Radiation Oncology; Gastro-Intestinal Oncology; and OB/GYN Oncology is concerned. That's a lot of bright minds. That's a lot of scary for us.

The plan, as of now, is to use very targeted high-dosage radiation on the tumor to shrink it (and provide pain relief, a very common theme between departments). We're told it's a "Cyber-Knife-like" treatment that will be given over the course of five days. Keep in mind that the Radiation Oncology doctor does not know what dosage the tumor will respond to. All he knows at this point is that low dosage will be ineffective (based on studies of previous unknown masses) and his targeting will be critical. Bones and nerves have a higher tolerance for radiation than intestines and organs, which the tumor has also involved itself with.

And the odds are high that there will be some bone or permanent nerve damage from this treatment.

After the series of high dosage treatments, Carole will be re-evaluated to see how the tumor responded. At that time, all options are on the table, including surgery to remove what can be removed safely, and chemo to remove what cannot be reached otherwise.

In other words, let's nuke it (intelligently) and see what happens. We are truly facing the unknown here.

THE PRAYER

In the meantime, we're planning on starting treatment as soon as they tell us they're ready. We have to handle logistics like transportation, housing and house-sitting, but all those are simple questions compared to the medical mystery that has thus far baffled Stanford University.

So, to all my atheist friends and readers, what would you do next? Who do you turn to for support? The old saying from WW II is that there are no atheists in foxholes. Now that the unknowns and uncertainties are dropping like bombs around us, how do you deal? Alcohol? I'm way ahead of you on that one, but nothing changes. If a medical crisis like this does not become a question of God (does He exist?), and for God (will He help?), then no question qualifies.

In summary, we're about to take a medical gamble, and we're not playing with house money.

So, for now, we're soaking up all this new information in a controlled state of shock, and asking God for mercy and compassion.

VACANCY

February 2, 2011

There is a run-down old motel along the highway just north of us. We pass it every trip to Stanford. It's still open, you can tell by how the cars change in the front, but it's not kept open by an exclusive clientele. No, in spite of its bright coral paint job, it's obvious that you don't need too much money to stay there. There is no HBO, no wifi, and no room service, just whatever you see when you open the door to the room, and I imagine that's not much. Some nights there are lots of cars there, some nights almost none, but the "Vacancy" sign is always lit.

The motel is VERY close to the highway, close enough for exceptionally convenient access to anywhere you want to go, and close enough so every car that passes shakes your bed, and reminds you that with any luck, this is not your destination, just a stop along the way.

Where is here? "Waiting".

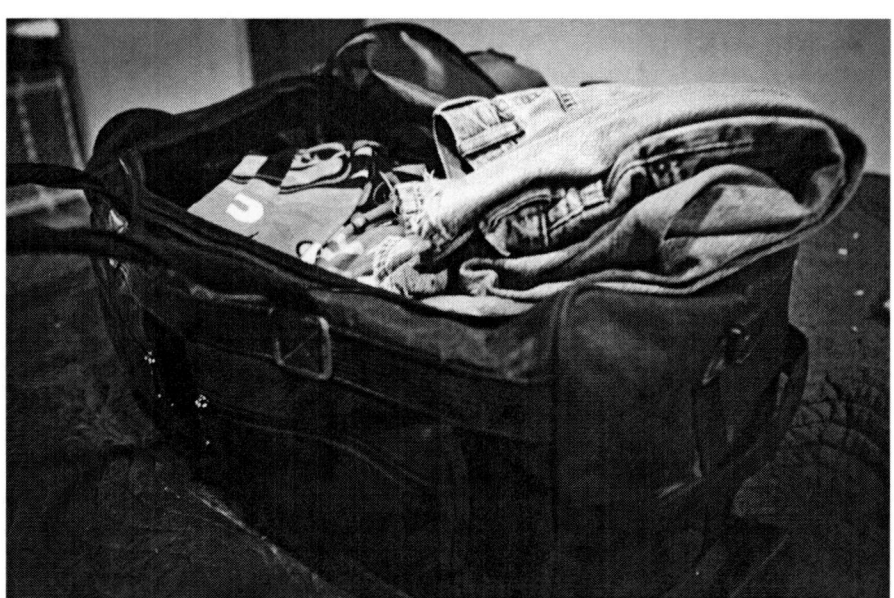

If your life had a GPS, you would find "Waiting" next to "Soon", in the state of "Uncertainty". You would also find many motels along the way like the one we're emotionally hunkered down in now.

We're in "Waiting" for Stanford to call so they can perform more scans, more tests, a "setup", and eventually radiation treatments. We're also in "Waiting" about what the insurance company has to say about all of this. Unknown details abound, but we're optimistic that all this will settle and we will be back on the road to Stanford "Soon".

We are not in the same emotional urgency as we were in when the pain was not controlled. No, there are days, and especially nights, when rest is possible, but the constant thunder from the highway still reaches our ears and reminds us that this is not the final resolution to all this. No, there is more travel, more treatments, more effort involved by everyone to get us to yet another "place of Uncertainty".

Ultimately, we'd like to find "Cure", but we may not be able to get there from here, since no one really knows where "Here" is, medically speaking. The doctors at Stanford speak from experience and with authority, but no one has yet found us on the map of medical way-points to "Cure". I'm sure we're in a familiar neighborhood, but no one else is "Here" to talk to.

So we rest and recharge, thankful that pain is better controlled, but aware this it is not completely "managed" yet. And we embrace the quiet, until the next car rolls by and shakes us out of our dreams, dreams brought on by exhaustion from the previous **months** of suffering and uncertainty.

And no life GPS can lead you to "Certainty". It either does not exist, or has not been discovered yet.

In either case, in our human condition we would all flock there if we could, and the motel sign out front would finally change to "No Vacancy".

Optimism and Fatigue

February 6, 2011

Things have been moving quickly. We didn't spend too many nights at that motel by the highway, thankfully, but we have reservations in another just like it.

Stanford was as good as their word, and called back with two appointments for today (Friday). This week we have been to Stanford twice, (at 330 miles per round trip) and to our local medical oncologist (once, but followed by a nice lunch and some quiet time together). In between all that fun was squeezed two days at the day job, and one night at the part-time job. What can I say? I've managed to stay out of trouble for five straight days, gotta be a record...

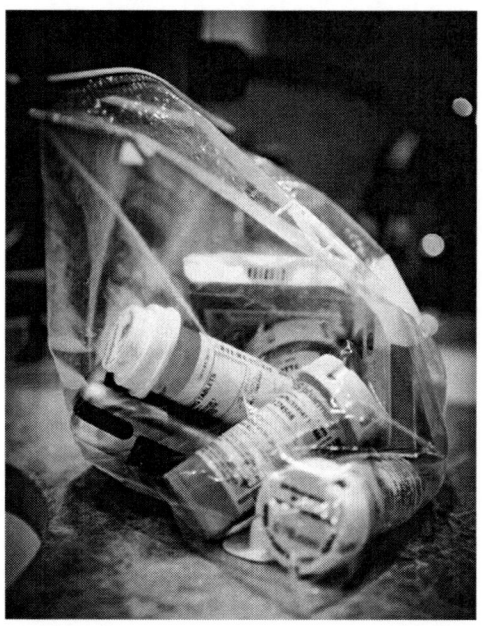

I confess right up front that I am a geek, but not a propeller-head (I don't live in Mom's basement). That said; I need to invoke the name of a propeller-head hero to explain what's about to happen to my wife in easy to understand scientific terms. So I hereby and humbly call upon the name of one of the greatest heroes of the basement dwelling, propeller-head sub-culture...Luke Skywalker.

Just about everyone on planet Earth has seen at least one Star Wars movie. Just in case you recently moved here from a galaxy far, far away, my summary of any Star Wars movie is this: various life forms run around the galaxy and eventually do battle. Why? Who cares, it's all about the tech toys. Everybody has his own starship, his own wardrobe, and his own weapons. For the record, my starship would have racing stripes and a wet bar. The stripes would imply speed and the wet bar would be for "sensitive" negotiations that happen often between intelligent, space travelling species. Everyone has stylish, deadly weapons, but the good guys have the coolest weapon of all, the Light Saber.

It seems that in every Star Wars episode, two life forms on opposite ends of the good guy/bad guy spectrum end up locked in a pose where they stand nose to nose, their Light Sabers crossed, hissing and popping with dramatic effect and color. This is clearly a power not to be trifled with.

Why do I invoke the name of a propeller-head god and his weapon du jour?

Because that's what is about to happen to my wife.

This new technology is called SBRT (affectionately referred to as "Saber"). In short, the radiologist will aim and fire multiple beams of radiation, like crossed Light Sabers, at Carole's tumor, and no one beam will do significant damage, but where they intersect will be blasted by a combined dose, a quantum dose. The delivery of these beams is so precise that surrounding tissues are spared damaging radiation, while the tumor gets nuked. In theory.

It's not a "Ready, Fire, Aim" technology. It requires accurate scans and medical physicists to come up with the coordinates. It also requires the patient getting a series of tattoos while in the CT scanner to calibrate the patient to the beams. That's what we did today. Yup, today we drove over 300 miles to the most expensive tattoo parlor in the world. Later this month those tattoos will be used much like a compass, guiding high-dose radiation to the same exact place five times over five days.

This treatment is a blessing on so many levels. No surgery, no chemo, no hair loss (for her), just radiation precisely targeted. Will this fix everything? No one knows. No one knows exactly what the tumor is, but most likely the tumor will be adversely affected by being lit up like Times Square on New Year's Eve. We hope that there will be change, but enough change to reduce pain and substantially increase her quality of life? Not sure. We know that there will be bone and nerve damage, but enough to affect her life permanently? Can't tell yet. The Cancer Casino is open, place your bets, drinks are free to gamblers like us.

There is also another, more pervasive element to all this; battle fatigue.

This battle started in October, it peaked in December and January as far as pain is concerned (just in time for the holidays), and will continue at least through the spring, if not all of 2011.

And frankly, the battle has changed us.

I have heard of "situational ethics", but what we sometimes experience in our house is "situational health". Today, if Carole can walk around the house without aid, then the day is defined as a good day. A good night is her only getting out of bed a half dozen times due to pain in her back, or her legs, or her guts.

Have I told you that I love to people watch? I do it everywhere, airports, malls, wherever people walk by. On our first visit to Stanford, while Carole was filling out the requisite paperwork, I watched patients come and go through the six cancer clinics. They all had one thing in common; they came and went under their own power. They may have been bandaged and even scarred, but they were alive, alive in the "I'm still fighting!" way. These were not survivors yet, but they were combatants, warriors, a band of brothers.

The old phrase goes "Fools go where angels fear to tread". We are in a place filled with anything but fools, surrounded by angels of all kinds, some even wearing white, but in spite of this new plan, this new weapon, this new optimism, there is a battle fatigue in this family. It lulls us into accepting a quiet day over a full life, a day of "managed" pain over painless days of the past. Yes, anyone in our situation should celebrate the little victories and quiet mercies, but not at the expense of losing the "big picture" view, the view of what life was like before war. This is the fatigue that I fight on a daily basis. This is the fatigue that sometimes quiets my writing voice, the "thousand yard stare" that clouds our vision of the past, and our expectations of the future.

We now have a plan, a weapon, an exact date and time of our attack, our enemy has been found and his position fixed. Now, it's about rest and regaining strength. Rest is a weapon, and hopefully it will restore our memory so we can recall the past and build a future that is more than "comfortable", more than "acceptable", and far more than it is now.

Tonight my wife will subject herself to narcotics more powerful than most people can endure and stay awake. Only people enduring the greatest of physical traumas can do this. I easily outweigh her by one hundred pounds and I would be on the floor from this dosage. Some call this impressive or sad, we call this "another night". (Note: I am finishing this post at 2:45 am on Sunday morning because Carole is having a bad night of pain, and I don't sleep well when my spouse is sobbing during what fitful sleep she can get. It's obvious her body is adjusting to the already new, higher level of pain meds.)

As grateful as we are for the prayers and thought of friends and family for comfort and rest, tonight we ask for prayers of fierce resistance, prayers of battle, prayers of survival against an enemy that has taken all our energy just to slow, not defeat. All these weeks have only redrawn the battle lines on a map, lines inside my wife on a scan, lines tattooed on her back, lines between pain and peace, past and future.

And we have moved on our own little map. We were in "Waiting", but we found ourselves briefly in "Progress". Now we're back in "Waiting" in the state of "Uncertainty", but closer to "Action" than we've ever been. "Uncertainty" is a big place.

The picture at the top of this post is her traveling bag of meds. It goes with her whether it's a 300+ mile trip or to the pharmacy to get more meds.

Hell On Wheels

February 8, 2011

A little over one hundred days ago she was a vibrant woman going to the doctor with a back ache. It literally feels like years ago, someone else's life ago. She tries to be the same person today, but her new body fails her so often and in so many ways.

We are back to "Waiting". Stanford and their high dosage radiation are only days away, but each day brings us so much change, and so much more challenge. Today, the wheelchair arrived. It's the product of another friend's compassion. There have been so many compassionate friends. The wheelchair will be used, regrettably, along with the new cane, and the additional medications.

No doctor will give us a prediction of life in one hundred days, and right now neither of us dare think that far. Our thoughts are limited in time and distance to the days and miles to Stanford. And radiation. And hope.

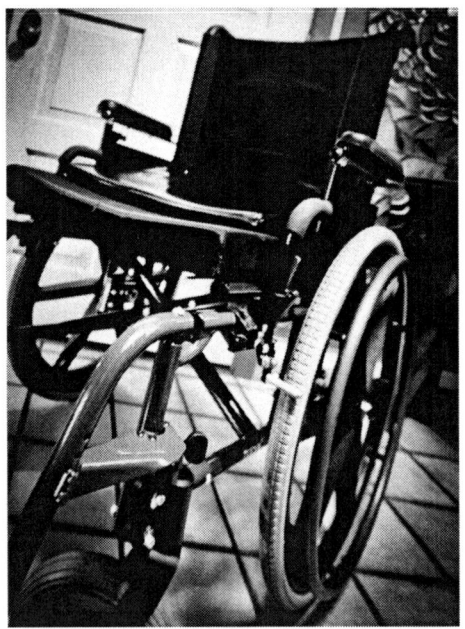

And that my friends, is now how we roll.

The Way We Were

February 9, 2011

Yeah, I know it's a song, but it's how I feel.

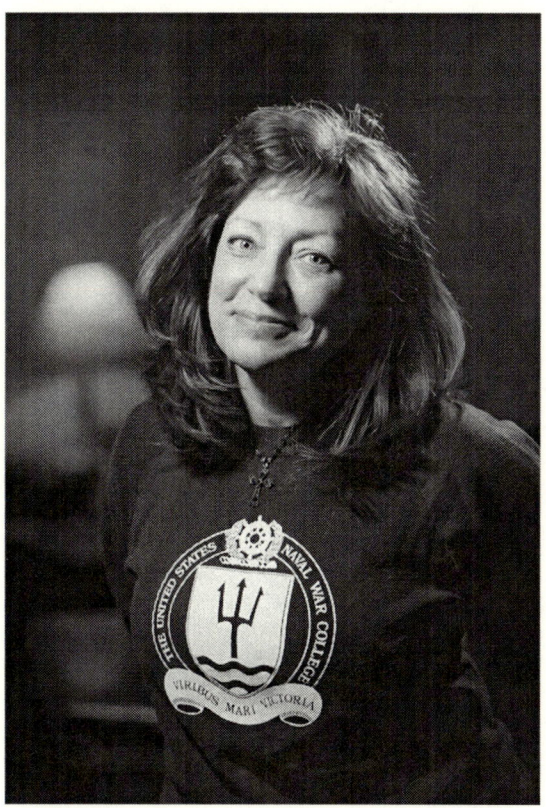

As recently as Halloween she was normal; her old self; independent, intelligent, sometimes ornery. She has a gift of linear thought and often she has to wait for me to come to the same conclusion, sometimes for days because I can be slow at times. OK, I'm slow.

What often got her most ornery is that I have an intuition that serves me well in things artistic. She earned everything in music because she worked her voice hard and paid her dues. I often got to skip to the head of the line because of a "gut" feeling or a good guess. She never really believed in my intuition until I picked up a camera and "translated" music into pictures. In spite of how it happened, she always supported me, always encouraged me to get off my ass and be better than I was. It's an understatement to say that whatever I am is because of her, whatever I am not is because of me.

As silly as it sounds, I knew her before I met her. I imagined such a woman so many times. I hoped that she existed, but never thought that someone like that would be interested in me. Ironically, I fell in love with her sight unseen. I heard her singing from another room before ever laying eyes upon her. She owned my heart before we met. Her voice was honey in my ears. When we were introduced she was a dream to my eyes, and her intelligence and sense of humor were far beyond mine. This was a life partner, a musical mentor, a teacher, a miracle, all wrapped in beauty. I was a dead man standing.

Her speaking voice has changed, her singing voice is gone, her humor only present in spurts when she has the energy, her legs betray her. I still love and respect her, but God I miss the old days.

I miss HER.

The picture at the top is of a patient life partner posing for yet another light test. Slow learners like me can only learn by experiment, and she was the willing test subject while I learned how to dial-in my small strobes. She has no make-up on, and is wearing my old navy sweatshirt, but this is what I am fighting to preserve, to restore. She's still in there; just trapped in a body that fails her at every turn.

I will not.

Sisyphus Meet Icarus

February 10, 2011

It would take TSA thirty minutes to inspect all of the bags under my eyes, and the airlines would charge me extra to fly with them. I don't understand this "sleep without rest" thing. Every morning feels like how I felt when I went to bed, all the same aches and pains, all the same worries, just less gas in the tank.

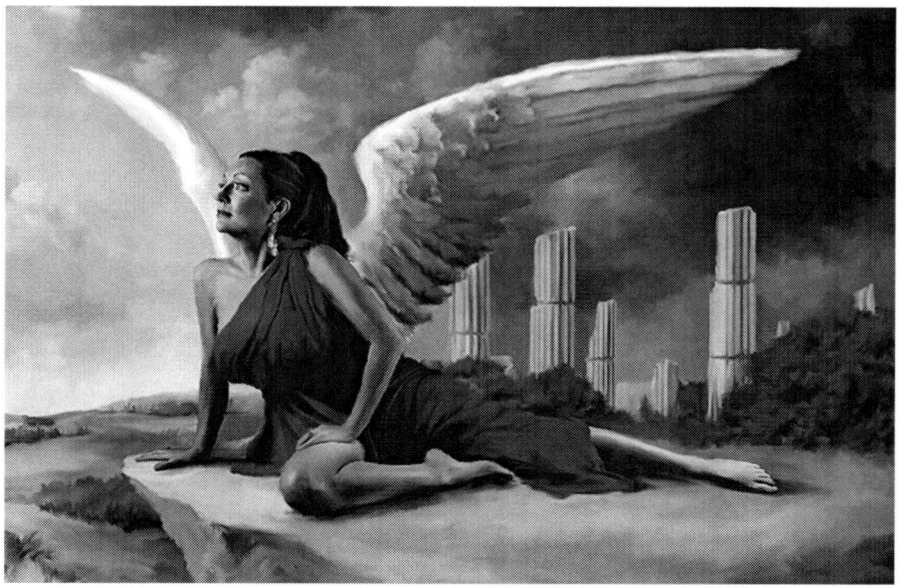

Digital Art by MichaelO www.bymichaelo.com

Strangely, (and I admit it, you can't spell "Bob" without "strange"), this reminds me of two ancient Greek legends. One guy (Sisyphus) lived a life of murder and robbery, and even tried to swindle the gods. His fate in the underworld was to roll a big rock up a big hill every day, just to see it roll down to the bottom every night. This was his sole purpose for eternity, rock and roll.

The second legend is Icarus, who, in spite of being warned not to fly too close to the sun with his wings of feathers and wax, did just that, and fell to his death into the sea. At least in his story, Icarus flew high enough to almost touch the sun. The freedom of that flight must have felt great (on the way up).

How do these legends relate to us?

A minute seems like a second to a drowning man (ask Icarus). It's the opposite for us. There is life, relief, and hope on the other side of this Stanford visit. Every day we see the sun travel the sky, and every day we try to push it along faster with our impatience. Our sole purpose, for what seems like an eternity, is to will the days by faster, until we are released from waiting, released to Stanford, and hopefully released from pain and worry. No, we don't expect a legendary cure in five days, but we do have hope for pain relief, and hope of more hope.

Until then, the alarm goes off at the same time every day, and it's back to work pushing the sun across the sky. Sisyphus, Icarus and Bob.

Sounds like a Rock and Roll band.

The picture at the top of the post is a digital creation by MichaelO (www.ByMichaelO.com), a friend of mine and a Fresno digital artist who has found the "big time" with his remarkable work. This work of his is based on a shot I took of Carole in 2007 (I think), and was a gift to her for Valentine's Day.

Fruitful Absurdity

February 14, 2011

Confession is good for the soul. That's the popular adage, one of the tenets of Christian theology, and probably part of every theology on earth. The self-inspection that comes before confession often bears fruit.

I have an unusual confession born from an extended period of self inspection. I hope this is good for my ragged, ragged soul, so here goes. I am fruitless, I am barren.

When I look inside myself, everything is gone. Everything I thought I knew is gone. Everything I hoped would happen is gone. Nothing is left but the dust and ash from the fire that I don't remember burning my core like tinder, and then like Dresden. And it's not just my wife's cancer.

Not one, not two, but three wonderful people in my life are each going through a private hell.

One is a young, vibrant, beautiful and generous woman with two perfect little girls who has recently endured a double mastectomy, and now endures chemo and later will endure radiation.

Another is an older, dignified, artistically gifted woman who recently had to admit to herself that caring for her husband of 50+ years, afflicted with Alzheimer's, was too much even for her love to conquer.

And, of course, my wife of brilliant mind and effortless integrity is enduring a cancer with no name and a treatment filled with risk, without a single guarantee of cure or comfort.

By all measures, my mind and soul should have imploded from all this weight weeks ago, months ago, but somehow, in spite of always being physically tired, I am prepared to lift ten times this emotional weight. Emotionally and spiritually I gain strength almost every day. I don't know how, but I know it happens.

To what can I credit this?

Absurdity.

THE CONFESSION CONTINUES

I have a college-age son. He lives on the east coast near his mom. His name is Ryan, and though he probably thinks differently about me, I am very impressed by him.

Oddly enough now, at this most personally challenging of times, my son referred me to a critical analysis of Sisyphus by Albert Camus. Yeah, I know it sounds very academic and almost incomprehensible, but it was appropriate, and perfect in its own way.

The point that Camus made was that enormous strength can come from weakness (and this is absurd by any logical definition). The short version is that if you love someone enough, you can stand by them even when they can't stand for themselves. It's nothing but a stubborn refusal to accept what your eyes see, and insisting on potential over prognosis. That stubbornness becomes strength. That strength is bottomless (so far). When loved ones are hurting so badly that it steals their energy, then you give them yours, and that gives you more. Absurd, but very, very real. (The side-effect from this is that you have little strength for the absurd minutia some people call their lives. Seriously, if Starbucks is out of Winter Blend, is suicide really an option? If so, please consider **ALL** your options carefully, and I take no responsibility for your actions, as well thought out as I know they'll be.)

Some would credit the source of this strength to faith, some to philosophy, but the strength is as real as your faith in that person, and my faith in these people is simply unshakable.

My kid taught me that, even though I knew it intuitively, sort of, maybe…or not. (There's that confession thing again).

And deep inside me, next to that seemingly bottomless well of strength, is a sapling of joy. How absurd is that? The help I can give my loved ones gives me a purpose, the most important purpose I've ever known. And these have been the most meaningful days of my otherwise exceptionally pointless life.

The love you have for others becomes strength. The weaker they become, the stronger you become, because you refuse to let the selfish universe rob you of people who are special, worth fighting for, remarkable even in their pain and weakness.

Some people I know will take their last breath and ask themselves if they got all they deserved. I hope to take mine asking if I gave all I could. This does not make me 'better' than another, it only means I measure my heartbeats on a different scale. (I will add a personal observation – if what you value has no value at a time like this, perhaps what you value is worthless.)

And the scale keeps tipping in my favor as more strength is added, and more stubbornness is added, and more caring is added.

The three people I care about will (hopefully) be whole again, especially if I can help them.

And as for the people I know who want everything they deserve, well, I hope they get everything they deserve.

Quantum Uncertainty

February 15, 2011

It's not like this whole adventure has been stepping from one certainty to another — it hasn't. The doctors aren't even certain what the tumor is, why should we have the luxury of certainty if they don't?

Just to fill you in, we were all emotionally prepared to start a five day course of very high-dose radiation targeted specifically at this tumor of unknown origin, when our Radiologist / Oncologist called on a Saturday and expressed second thoughts. He had been in consultation with colleagues all over the country, but a colleague at Harvard convinced him that if the patient (Carole) was in a wheelchair now (she is), then the nerve damage done by the radiation would strand her there, for life. It would probably kill the tumor, but the collateral damage would be to the nerves running down to her lower extremities. These are the very same nerves under siege right now.

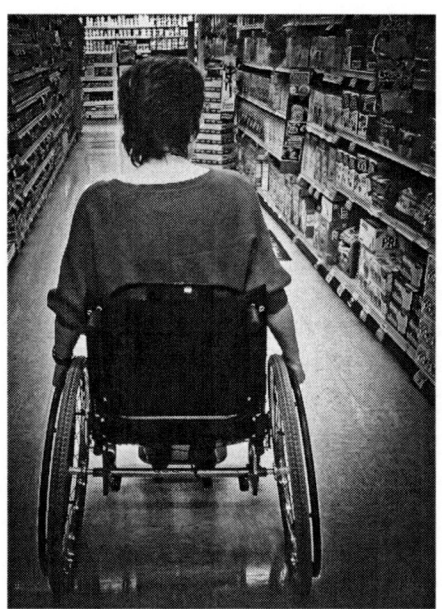

To our doctor's credit, he could not condone that.

He first proposed a lower-dose radiation course over eight weeks, and then five weeks. Please note, this course of radiation is **FIVE DAYS A WEEK** for five to eight weeks in a hospital 160 miles away. When I asked him if anyone locally (to Fresno) could administer his "prescription", his answer was that it was unfair to ask another colleague to assume the high-risk this treatment entailed.

So Stanford Radiology it is, or was, until he called back and explained that he found a neurosurgeon on staff willing to explore the case. Yup, new plan. Now we're going to Stanford on Monday so a neurosurgeon can run pre-surgical scans, and decide if he can go where so far angels, and our Fresno surgeon, have dared not tread.

The plan by our Radiologist is very simple and compassionate: get that tumor away from those nerves, and I'll blast it to next Tuesday without putting her in a wheelchair for life. It's up to the neurosurgeon to decide if he can get in there, pick out the tumor from the nerves, get out, and leave Carole walking.

In the meantime, we prepare for eight weeks of radiation, five weeks of radiation, surgery, no surgery, wheelchair for life, wheelchair for 2011, no wheelchair. If there is such a place as the far side of God's love, we're there. We're both feeling emotionally exhausted and spiritually flat. If the cavalry is supposed to charge over the hill, then now is the time.

Any time you're ready. Anytime now. Hit it, bugler.

And our insurance company is reeling from the changes. They already denied an MRI requested by Radiology to better target the tumor, since an MRI had recently been done in Fresno. (Not of the exact same area of the body, but so what?) On top of that, I literally just got off the phone with Stanford, saying that I would pay for the as-yet-not-approved-by-the-insurance-company-MRI that the neurosurgeon is requesting. What am I supposed to do, tell him to make due with the previous scans? I have no idea what he needs or whether it's valuable to him or not.

All I do know is that my wife is in a wheelchair today, and probably will be tomorrow, and the day after that until a plan is agreed upon, acted upon, and the damage assessed.

A vital, independent, intelligent woman's quality of life hangs in the balance, and money is not going to stop me from restoring her to the best Stanford can do.

(Insurance companies and hospitals can take my car, my house, and my retirement, but they'll never be able to slap the smile off my face when she walks into their office and shows them what they declined to pay for.)

Honestly, we're both exhausted. If we could will our hearts to stop and join God in heaven together right now, we would, but the truth is that we can't, and we don't know what the course of treatment will be, if she will walk again, or what zip code our next meal will be in. We're at the mercy of Stanford's expertise, and Stanford's mercy.

The picture at the top of this post was taken today as we shopped for the unknown amount of food needed for the unknown length of stay 160 miles away for an unknown course of treatment with a non-guaranteed outcome.

If that doesn't define life, then nothing does.

The Road Ahead

February 16, 2011

This morning I was greeted by dark, foreboding clouds outside. It wrapped our little town like a blanket, and just made me all-the-more aware how much I wanted to be inside, in my bed, wrapped in my own warm blanket, instead of packing the car for another trip to Stanford. I must admit that I am getting better and better at it with all the practice. We now have a new addition to our 'road pack', a portable wheelchair. That's in addition to the other wheelchair we were given to use for the duration. In fact, we had a third wheelchair offered to us, but we politely refused. There is a thin line between giving Carole her freedom and turning the house into a used car lot. (Ironically, she has put very low mileage on them and she only uses them for trips to the market and church.)

As we headed out, the skies opened up and a deluge of rain hit us. It was one of those "biblical" downpours where you could actually imagine floods and arks. My thought at the time was, "So what, we've been through so much already, we can handle it. One more plague might actually go unnoticed."

Strangely, as we turned to the west, the clouds began to blow away, the sun came out, and a rainbow was in front of us – and not just any rainbow! It started as a small splash of color on the horizon, and eventually grew to look like a paint factory on fire. The colors were billowing out from the ground and seemed to blow away. It was so large and vibrant that, for a while, we thought we would be able to touch it over the next hill.

Very intense color? Yes. Very intentional message? I'll get back to you on that.

(BTW, the rainbow in Scripture is God's promise to Noah that He won't flood the earth again. I wouldn't want anyone to miss the point of all this typing).

Our conversation in the car started out light. I was able to make her laugh pretty often, but then her mood, much like the roads we were travelling, began to change. Her bravery, her fear, her exhaustion, her hopes all went up and down, like the hills we were driving through.

It is now 12:15 pm. We have been at this Stanford imaging center for about an hour. Her first scan is done, and she's in having her second one now. At 3:00 pm, we will see the neurosurgeon to get his "opinion" on if this is an operable tumor, if he can save her from the pain that exists in her every breath, and whether he can reduce the odds that her wheelchair becomes permanent.

Don't worry, the hospital is only 4.5 miles away according to the GPS, we'll make the appointment with time to spare.

But it's going to be one of the longest roads we've ever driven.

Today, Tomorrow, Friday, Forever

February 19, 2011

This is what happened. This is how it felt.

WEDNESDAY

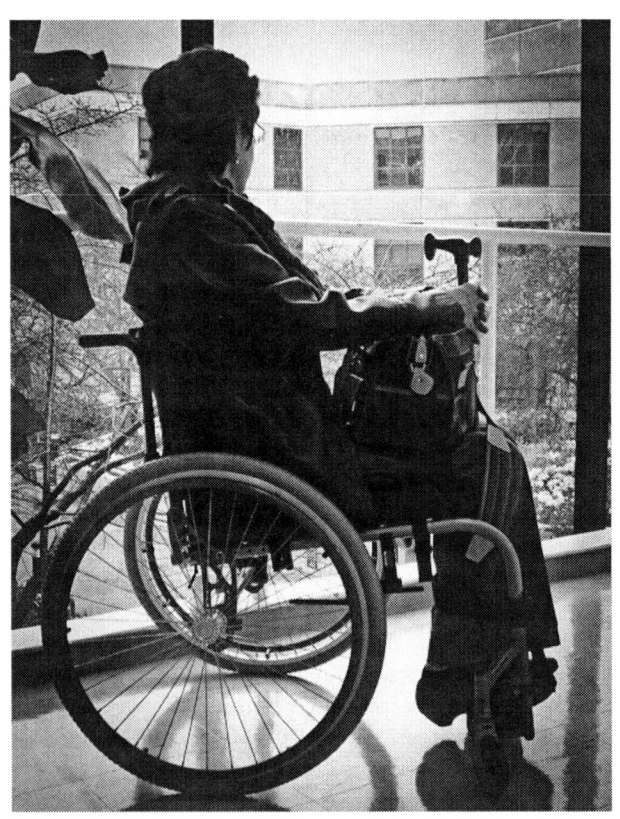

BOB MARCOTTE

The appointment with the neurosurgeon was, to his credit, brutally honest. He spoke in bold, declarative sentences, but each sentence landed like a freight train on our ears and hearts.

Yes, it's operable, but at a high cost.

The best we can hope for is your current condition, perhaps less.

To get to the tumor I need to remove your sacrum and replace it with titanium rods.

We remove the tumor 'en bloc', in one piece, but that requires getting to it, removing every visible trace of it, and then plastic and vascular surgeons rebuild what is left.

The surgery will most likely take eighteen hours, and a team of me and three more surgeons whom I trust and respect.

The nerve disability that now weakens your legs will be permanent, since I will cut those nerves when I remove your sacrum. They weren't coming back anyway.

Recovery is two weeks in the hospital followed by one agonizing year of pain and physical therapy.

No, you won't be released home from the hospital, you'll be released into a 24/7 physical therapy facility. There you will learn to live with what physical limitations you have and what physical abilities you have left.

We will follow this up with a course of radiation to kill what microscopic cancer cells remain.

Do you want to live two years or twenty years? Yes, you will be in a wheelchair but at least you'll be alive.

We took turns being strong, but Carole was silenced early in the "conversation". I took the point, and asked a handful of semi-intelligent questions before I too succumbed to the magnitude of what it was we had heard. We needed time to process, time to accept the unacceptable, to come to grips with our worse fears.

My wife, who sat mute in her borrowed wheelchair, just heard the words that put her in that chair until her last heartbeat and I could not do a fucking thing about it. I asked God for a replay, surely I had heard something wrong – but no, this was reality under God's mercy, on His watch.

Out of the deep I cried on deaf ears. This was our reality and our religion rolled into one plea, one denied plea for mercy.

We finished the appointment with polite discussion about prescriptions, but we were both in shock, both needing a quick escape from the Stanford of our optimism to a place we could just be alone and process it all. Before we left, we committed to making a phone call to the surgeon the next morning telling him if we were in or out of his plan. He gave us a night to "sleep" on it. A thirty-minute drive to the dive motel we could afford allowed us the space we needed, but we both heard the same things. Neither of us could deny nor explain away what we had heard.

Wheelchair, permanent, rehab, pain, more pain than now, a full year, lots of fentanyl for pain, years versus months.

I would have given her my spare parts to spare her from this gauntlet. In fact, kill me now and take the parts you need while they're still warm.

WEDNESDAY NIGHT

Over a dinner of "comfort food", she said repeatedly that I hadn't signed on for this. Fine print I joked, it was in the fine print, next time I'll know better. Then she started a sentence with, "You know..." Before she could finish I answered, "Yes." I know what we're facing; yes I have a good idea of the emotional cost, yes. But no, I will not leave you alone.

Business-like conversation and gallows humor filled in the time during dinner. Since her driving days are over, we need to sell her little blue car, the one that matches her eyes. I also volunteered to sell my car since what we need is an SUV capable of stowing a wheelchair, among other things. We also dreamed about a motorcycle with sidecar so we could both ride the hills around home with the people we enjoyed, and a handicap-accessible motor home.

That night she tossed and turned in an uncomfortable, over-medicated sleep in this fleabag motel, while I wrote this through tears, but nothing has really changed. I WILL be there for her. Today. Tomorrow. A year from tomorrow. Nothing's changed.

And I will be filling my spare time with some very honest, sometimes highly disrespectful conversations with God about my wife's present and future suffering. I will most likely over-imbibe and end up on the floor tonight, but Lord God, maker of heaven and earth; I will save you some confusion. I may be on my knees soon but it has nothing to do with thanks and praise. It has to do with buckling under today's events and feeling quite outside the mercy you're renowned for.

Tomorrow we inform friends and family. Tomorrow we drive home, since Stanford has no use for us. Tomorrow I take Advil for the headache, but nothing changes. Tomorrow is for us just another day with cancer, but a day totally dedicated to mulling over the cost of survival.

THURSDAY DAY AND NIGHT

We took our time on Thursday morning. We talked things over and we agreed on three things: first, that the way things were now was unacceptable. Second, surgery followed by radiation was the best and only option to remove the cancer once and for all, and third, it was ultimately Carole's decision. In her mind, this was a no-brainer, so a call was made to the surgeon saying we were on for surgery. He took the call himself, and stated that using just radiation on a tumor this big was like trying to put out a three alarm fire with a bottle of Evian.

He advised us to stand by for a series of phone calls for required pre-surgical tests that he hoped to get done while we were still in the area.

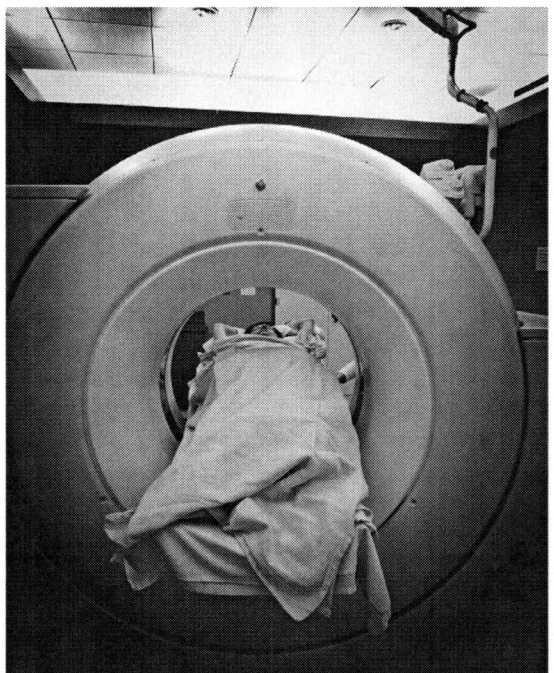

True to his word, the phone rang just minutes later, and we were scheduled for another CT scan (at yet another Stanford location) for 12:30. That test went quietly with the typical charming and caring Stanford staff (thank you Wendy and David!) and then it was back to the hotel for more talk, perhaps a nap and dinner at Appleby's. It was a humble plan.

Close to 5 pm the phone rang, it was the GI Oncologist. She was telling us to get to the Stanford Emergency Room right now. I requested the phone and asked the doctor to repeat herself. What Carole had heard as "lung spots" (a condition we knew about since the scans in Fresno) was actually "blood clots" in her lungs. Pulmonary emboli to you trained readers out there. Our evening of rest was broken up by a four hour adventure in the Stanford Hospital Emergency Room. Eventually the Doc prescribed a VERY small shot to be self-administered every twelve hours to contain the blood clots and prevent more from forming.

Yes, the Doctor was technically correct that a Pulmonary Embolism is not to be treated lightly, but the already physically and emotionally exhausted patient did not need the additional stress or the physical effort required of an ER visit. It entailed going through a metal detector, having her handbag searched, and answering the same questions over and over, including the one that makes us laugh now, "Are you in any pain?"

It was magnified by the college-aged girl in the next bed screaming for pain meds. When asked how bad her pain was on a scale from one to ten, she answered, "thirty". Before and after her pain shot, she and her girlfriend continued their discussion of restaurants in "the city", and their next dinner date in whispered tones, while Carole, on fentanyl patches, fentanyl pops, and Norco to handle the break-through pain, lay stoically in the next bed, offended and disgusted by the folly. I admit that I was interested in introducing the spoiled princess in the next bed to a REAL pain level of thirty on more than one occasion (especially when she referred to her father as "Daddy", as in, "Daddy works in the city, and knows all the best places to go,"). Personally, it would have been an act of joy, not violence, and a real stress-reducer.

In this ER, the person who screamed the loudest and put on the best show got her candy the fastest. However, the attending physician in the ER was onto their game, and made them wait for their test results, in spite of their complaints every fifteen minutes, and their threats to go "over his head".

Thanks to that same attending physician, we were eventually discharged and our dinner plans ended up being a drive-through burger since by this time Carole was weeping from the yesterday's news, the stress of the ER, and pain.

We fell asleep in each other's arms, crying ourselves to sleep.

FRIDAY

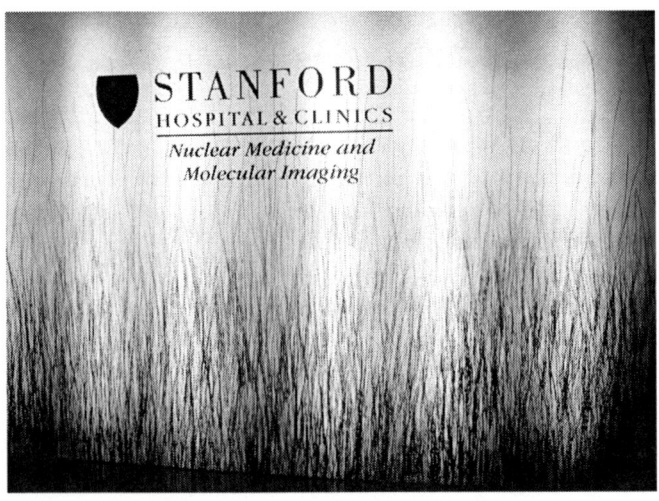

Friday we had only one test scheduled, the PET scan. Unfortunately, the usual level of Stanford care was missing. Once Carole was dressed in the typical gown, and was comfortable, I volunteered to go to the Cancer Clinic and pick up the prescription from last night, and another that we had asked to be renewed. The building is across the courtyard, and it was raining outside. I was trying to prevent her from getting cold and wet.

While I was gone, Carole was literally forgotten and abandoned. It was so bad that the doctor tasked with giving her an injection to be traced by the scan "forgot" that she was there. Once his busy mind was refreshed, it cost us an additional hour at the Nuclear Medicine clinic and Carole spent the time in tears. I have noticed that she has abandonment issues lately, and who could blame her? In a building with literally ten thousand souls, is it too much to ask that someone remember the patient in room one?

In the meantime, I finally caved-in to the weight I had been carrying around since Wednesday. This was the first opportunity to be away from Carole for an extended time since "the news", and I broke down badly. In the middle of a phone call to my boss describing the last few days' events, I started weeping and could not stop. I thought I was strong enough to describe the prognosis over the phone, but I was fooling myself. I found an out-of-the-way passage between buildings and wept like a child, asking God for mercy and more mercy. The cold Stanford rain met the warm tears on my cheeks as I finally vented what I had needed to vent since the appointment with the surgeon on Wednesday.

The answer to my tears did not take long. I was asked by security to "move along". Someone in one of the offices must have reported me as a psycho patient off his meds making a scene.

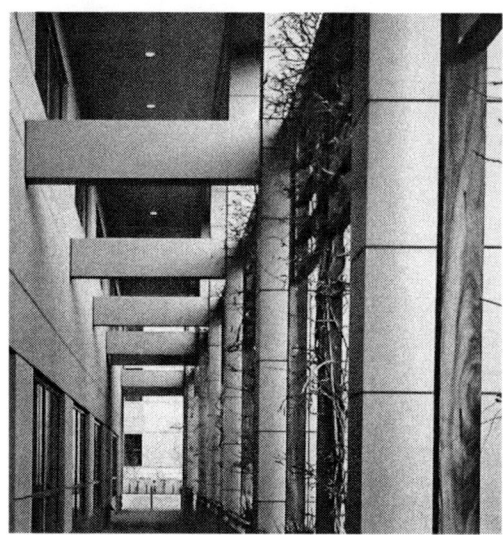

Just to "serve and protect" the good citizens and patients of Stanford, the guard followed me at a respectful distance while I got the meds Carole needed at the pharmacy and walked back to the hospital in the rain, to start our journey home and to a whole new life.

PLAYDAYS

February 20, 2011

So, after three days of Stanford, we finally got our wish and spent Friday night in our own home. It was like being inside castle walls for us. We felt like we belonged here and we were protected.

Saturday morning came right on schedule for us (like it did for you), and over coffee we decided that everything, and nothing, had changed. We fell back on an old adage we had used in on our theater and jazz combo days, "if it's not tested, it's broken". If this was truly what our future held, then let's get outside, into life, and practice how we're going to get around, how we're going to navigate this new world. I loaded up the "big" wheelchair into our trusty Montero (the one with 117,000 miles on it), and we ventured out for a day of typical errands that every family in the United States seems to do on any given Saturday.

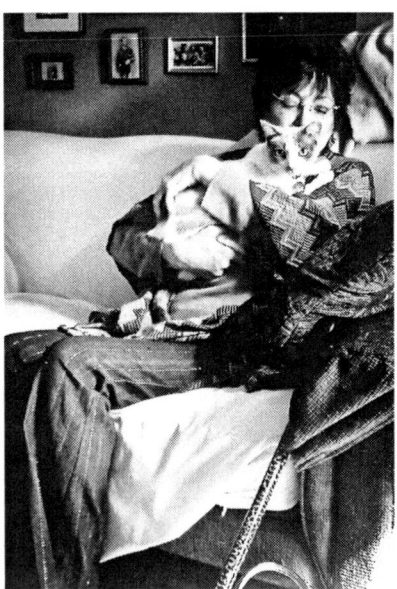

On our first errand I packed the wheelchair wrong and one of the wheels spun the entire time we were in motion. I made an adjustment for our second trip that stopped the wheel, but now the chair was spinning during the trip. By trip number three, I had both chair and wheel under control, and now we were committed to enter the one store that brings fear to every male in America – Bed, Bath and Beyond.

I admit to being clueless as to what they sell, but the way they stack it up to the ceiling and into the aisles is very claustrophobic for me. This time, we had the strategic advantage. Even the most stubborn bargain shopper will move for a woman in a wheelchair (as long as they both aren't staring at the same sale item). With few exceptions, we could navigate where we wanted to go. It was like being the captain of an estrogen icebreaker, parting the way for others behind us to find the most perfect bathroom accessories known to humankind. This was freedom; this was mastery of the seas. Like a hot knife through butter, we went everywhere and cashed out in record time. Score one unexpected point for the wheelchair.

But a thought did come to mind while wandering through all the "sale" tags and "reduced for quick sale" price tags. We are now living in a world where money no longer exists. No, I'm not quitting my job, but if you pretend that we won the largest lottery in U.S. history, does that change anything? Is having a wheelchair with GPS and seven drink holders enough compensation for the pain and the life-altering change of an unknown cancer? Don't get me wrong, if I had the opportunity I would get her the biggest Lazy-Boy on wheels ever made if it were comfortable for her, but the only value in it would be her comfort. Money has ceased to have value if it brings no comfort or security to Carole, period.

We tried to live as "normal" a life as we could, including checking in on our friend's pets while they were away as we had promised. As is typical, all the pets gravitated to Carole, including the elusive cat who jumped into her lap and tolerated hugs, kisses and whispered secret messages. She only became suspicious when I broke out my cell phone to take pics so the owners would believe us.

All in all, we proved to ourselves that life will not stop because of a wheelchair. We are, however, still dealing with the idea that we are not "playing", that this is, in fact, a change that will last "forever".

Because

February 20, 2011

All kidding and light-hearted adventures aside, the idea that my most precious loved one has to go through hell to come out (potentially) cancer-free is a tough thought to accept. Here is a woman that I completely respect, and in so many ways admire, who has been told that she has to go through the purifying fire of pain to stay among us. It's just not fair. She inhales more integrity reading a book than some people I know breathe in a day, a week, or a lifetime, she doesn't deserve this.

My sole purpose, as I understand it now, is to push her wheelchair, in her broken state, to the very gates of hell. My purpose is to help her push open those gates and endure the trip out the other side. As undeserving as she is, as incomplete as she has become, my job is to run as hard as I can and get her through hell as fast as I can, so she can endure life in a new way, in a compromised way, with a survivor's acceptance. I'd prefer to put a gun to my head and pull the trigger than to have to do this to her, but if I am worth even a single breath in my meaningless life, I will do this.

I don't look forward to seeing Satan in person. I don't look forward to feeling the heat of hell on my face, and seeing the pain on hers, but I will do this. I would give my very body to be beaten and burned for her, but I will do this.

I feel like such a traitor that I am the one who will drive her to Stanford, to escort her to such a fate. Who but the most sadistic among us would do such a thing?

But I will.

I will drag her soul through hell knowing her body will not survive intact, because her soul is worth it, because her intelligence and integrity are worth it.

Because I am given no choice.

Because I love her.

CONVERSATIONS

February 24, 2011

It's been a week since our "conversation" with the surgeon. For the record, it could barely be called a conversation. He spoke, we just held our breath.

Both of us are an emotional pendulum – some hours we're strong, some hours we're scared. It just keeps swinging back and forth.

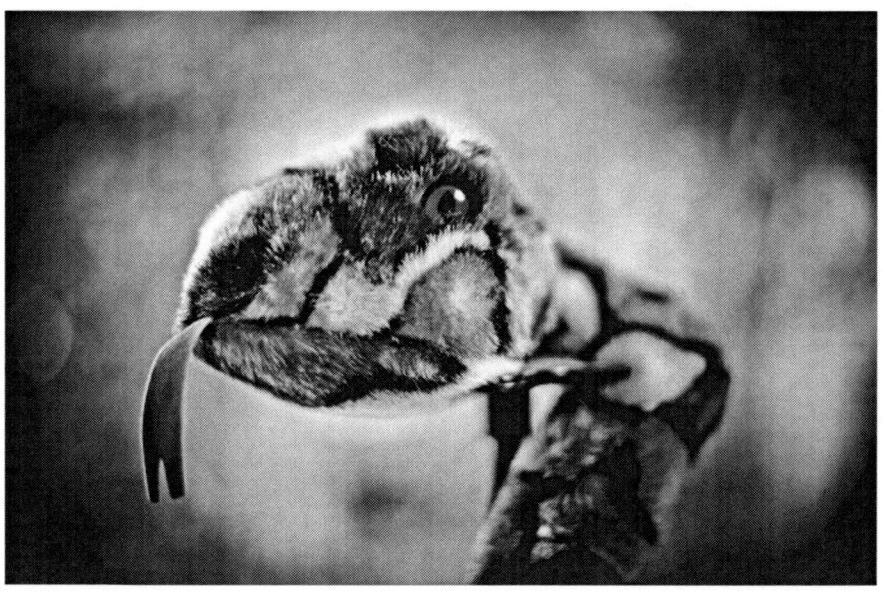

And we're also jumpy every time the phone rings. Just a few minutes ago it rang and it was Stanford surgery returning my call. No, we don't have a set surgery date yet, but it will be in early March, "hang in there".

"Hang in there". Yeah, like we have a choice, hang in there we will, but time and silence are a very potent pain unto themselves nowadays. After all the tests and examinations and appointments of last week, the silence of this week is intimidating.

You get a sense of this kind of anxious silence at Stanford, just not as intensely. There are knowing glances between patients in waiting rooms, silent conversations. Total strangers now bonded by a common struggle will sit wordlessly, everyone needing the support of one another, but no one willing to break the silence and intrude. But the conversations cannot be stopped. So, how are you handling the pain? You can't sleep either? Where's your tumor? What kind is it? Do you always have that funny taste in your mouth from the meds? How much painkiller are you on? It's finally time for my appointment, but I wish you the very best of luck and sometimes a "God Bless You".

"God Bless You". Yeah, that was right up there with "hang in there", until recently.

There was another, not so silent conversation last Thursday, the morning after the "conversation" with the surgeon. I was awakened not by Carole or the smell of coffee. Everything was unusually still, except for a repeating whisper. It said to me "This is not my doing. Do you really think I would have allowed cancer in the Garden of Eden?" As soon as I was awake enough to realize what was happening, it was gone. I begged, "Please come back, we need you!", but there was nothing. Just silence, not unlike the silence we're experiencing now.

Of course, that put my puny little brain into overdrive for the last week, and this is what I came up with...

If it wasn't God, then it must have been that other guy.

Shopping for Joy

March 7, 2011

OK, now is the time for another very personal confession. In fact, I have spoken of this to only one person in my life — my wife. Surprisingly, she hasn't had me committed — yet.

When I am in the worlds I belong in, the worlds of feelings, such as music and photography, I have a catalog of feelings within me that I can refer to as needed. I remember anguish and bliss in the same amount of detail. When I need to play "sad", I have an emotional memory of "sad" that is as exact and full as I can possibly contain. The same goes for love, happiness, sorrow and satisfaction.

I remember the layers of joy and doubt that make up each emotion. I can call upon those feelings as needed to play not only the feeling I need, but the *shades* of feeling I need. Think of it as a painter choosing the perfect shade of blue to describe his sadness. Carpenters cut wood to exacting length; artists cut emotion to the exact depth. This catalog is in my soul.

Recently, my wife wanted to shop in a store going out of business. The card we received in the mail advertised up to 90% off. This is an event my wife cannot dismiss even in her existing condition, it's a part of her very DNA, and it brings her great joy. The part that caught me unprepared was watching her shop in her wheelchair.

She struggled as she pushed her way through the aisles crowded with racks of clothes. Sometimes she had to push the clothes back to make room for her and her chair. The effort was enormous for her weakened body, especially since she could muster no leverage from her seated position. She will never stand and shop again; she will never be able to see the price tags eye to eye. Yeah, there are much bigger issues in play right now, but this is just one of the simple joys of her life that just got very, very complicated.

Take my piano, hell, take my hands and I will deal with it, but my heart breaks watching my wife do what she enjoys doing so much in such a compromised fashion. While she struggled through the store, I struggled with holding back tears. Her joy, in fact her life was compromised, and therefore, so was mine.

Nothing in my selfish little catalog of emotions prepared me for this. Compromising so many elements of her life to preserve our life together is new territory for both of us, and watching the change is painful and profound for me. I can't imagine what it's like for her.

This is life now, and after surgery this will be life forever.

My soul is filled with tears today, but I'll take it. We will make the changes required to give her a life as full as anyone else's, wheelchair be damned.

And as we figure this whole thing out, I will redefine many of the emotions in my catalog, especially the sad ones, as we redefine the rest of our lives. Eventually I hope to define a brand new emotion for the catalog as I watch her overcome and adapt.

Pride.

IF

March 9, 2011

by Rudyard Kipling

If you can keep your head when all about you
   Are losing theirs and blaming it on you;
If you can trust yourself when all men doubt you,
   But make allowance for their doubting too;
If you can wait and not be tired by waiting,
   Or, being lied about, don't deal in lies,
Or, being hated, don't give way to hating,
   And yet don't look too good, nor talk too wise;
If you can dream – and not make dreams your master;
   If you can think – and not make thoughts your aim;
If you can meet with triumph and disaster
   And treat those two imposters just the same;
If you can bear to hear the truth you've spoken
   Twisted by knaves to make a trap for fools,
Or watch the things you gave your life to broken,
   And stoop and build 'em up with wornout tools;
If you can make one heap of all your winnings
   And risk it on one turn of pitch-and-toss,
And lose, and start again at your beginnings
   And never breath a word about your loss;
If you can force your heart and nerve and sinew
To serve your turn long after they are gone,
And so hold on when there is nothing in you
Except the Will which says to them: "Hold on";
If you can talk with crowds and keep your virtue,
   Or walk with kings – nor lose the common touch;
If neither foes nor loving friends can hurt you;
   If all men count with you, but none too much;
If you can fill the unforgiving minute
   With sixty seconds' worth of distance run -
Yours is the Earth and everything that's in it,
And – which is more – you'll be a Man my son!

Waiting Redefined

March 12, 2011

This started at Halloween, appropriately enough. It's not going to end soon, but it will change. Change for the better? Can't say. Sacrificing bones and organs for more heartbeats is only better if you make those heartbeats worthwhile. That's one of my future jobs.

Today, yesterday, and last week, all I've been doing is to help coordinate the mountain of appointments and tests my wife needed to attend to before surgery. It's much like a tour through a company as a new employee. We had to check in with each surgeon, let him explain what his portion of the surgery is, and sign the consent form. (For the record, there may be as many as seven surgeons involved over the course of the two scheduled surgeries.). At each appointment, we were greeted with the "*so you're the one*" greeting. Lucky game show winners know what I'm talking about. Each surgeon politely concealed his "interest" in the case, the kind of interest that put him into medicine in the first place. Yes, these professionals were all caring and compassionate but their questions were all the same, "*when did this start?*", "*when did you notice?*", "*what was the diagnosis in 2003, 2006, 2010, now?*" They seemed to be thinking, "*satisfy my curiosity, I've only read about this condition in books, I may never see this again in my lifetime*".

And at each stop we either had our optimism raised or smashed. I had been carrying a quiet hope that perhaps part of the sacrum could be saved. Nope, the cancer is also in the bone so it all goes. Ironically, I was pessimistic about the right kidney but we were told that they think they can save it. After each appointment we reset our emotional expectations and moved on. It's a cruel experience, but we've had so much practice that we really do just move on.

In all cases, the last thing before the "*see you at surgery*" farewell was the signing of the consent form. Previously, I had defined "consent" as having a part in making a choice. Believe me; the suffering she is fighting through daily gives her no choice. Who would sign a form allowing surgeons to remove organs, bowels and bones if she actually had a choice not to?

Her last procedure was done yesterday. It was the insertion of an IVF filter which is supposed to stop blot clots from getting stuck in some really important places like the heart and the brain. The procedure does not take that long, but it did give me more practice at waiting, (like I really need more practice at waiting.)

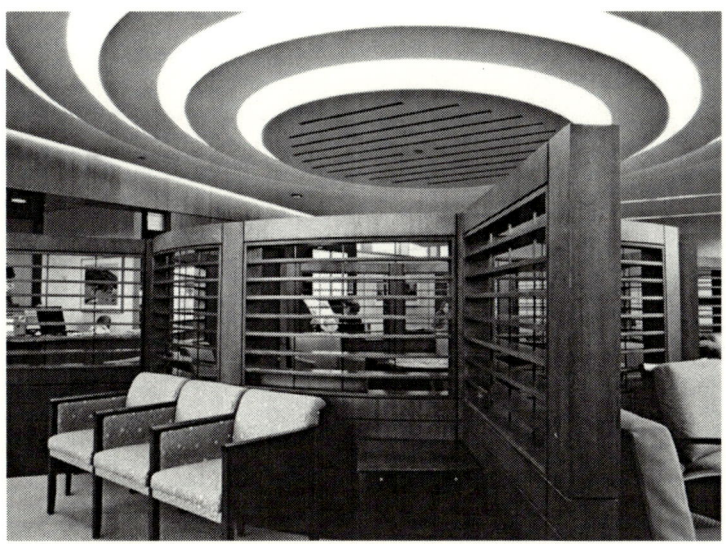

What I'm starting to notice as we get closer and closer to surgery are the unique Stanford touches for those who wait. The staff is overwhelming in their humanity, their people skills always seem so genuine, and they're so willing to answer questions and share information. The not knowing is the hardest part of the waiting, and Stanford really does try to keep the family in the loop.

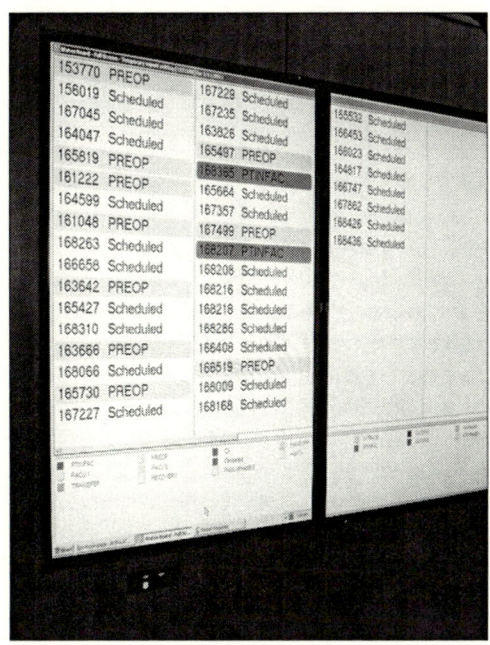

But regardless of how they try to avoid it, everyone who passes through the "staff only" doors gets redefined. You are redefined by medical record number, case number, your birth date and your belongings. Colorful wristbands are attached to each patient to identify allergies to medications, pre-existing conditions and any special warnings (such as fall risk).

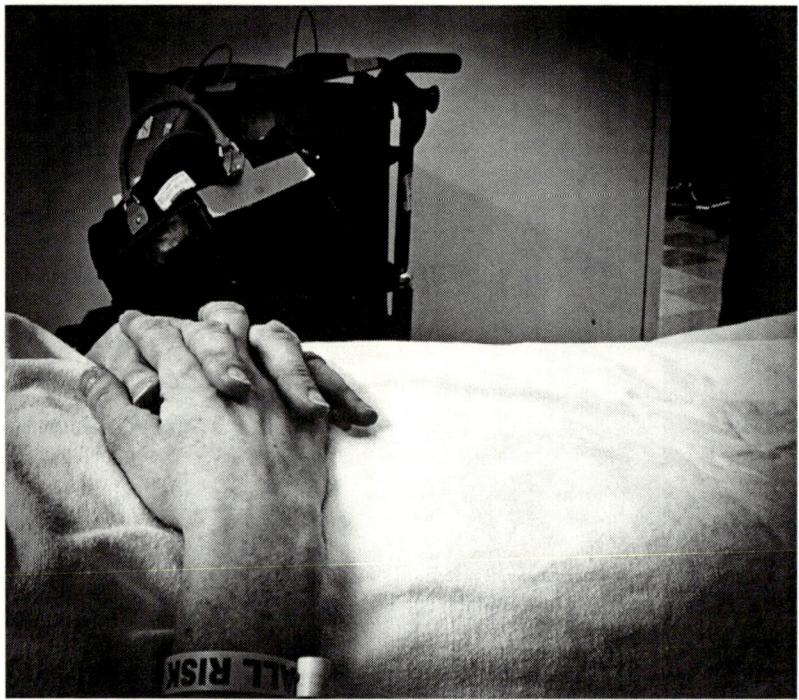

I was taken aback by how much Carole has been redefined since Halloween. How her recent life can be summed up by a few wristbands, her cane, her wheelchair, a handbag filled with pain meds and a paper bag of clothes. Nothing there tells the story of her suffering, there is nothing marking her strength and bravery.

It is said that the body cannot remember pain. Let it also be said that spouses do. These very long months of waiting for diagnosis, testing and a plan have been unbearable for her, yet she endured. Something as common as a night's sleep has become commonly inhumane. When I took the picture above, I wished that I could give her a wristband that said "Tough As Nails", or "Respect This Patient Above Others – She Has Suffered Greatly to Get This Far". It's not that the Stanford staff disrespects anyone, but the military gives out medals for far less than this, companies gives out employee of the year plaques for less than this, I just wanted the medical professionals to know that she is well on her way through hell and she will come out the other side. I just wanted someone else to know her story besides me. I just wanted someone else to show her the respect she deserves besides me.

I have added that to my new list of jobs I've taken on since Halloween.

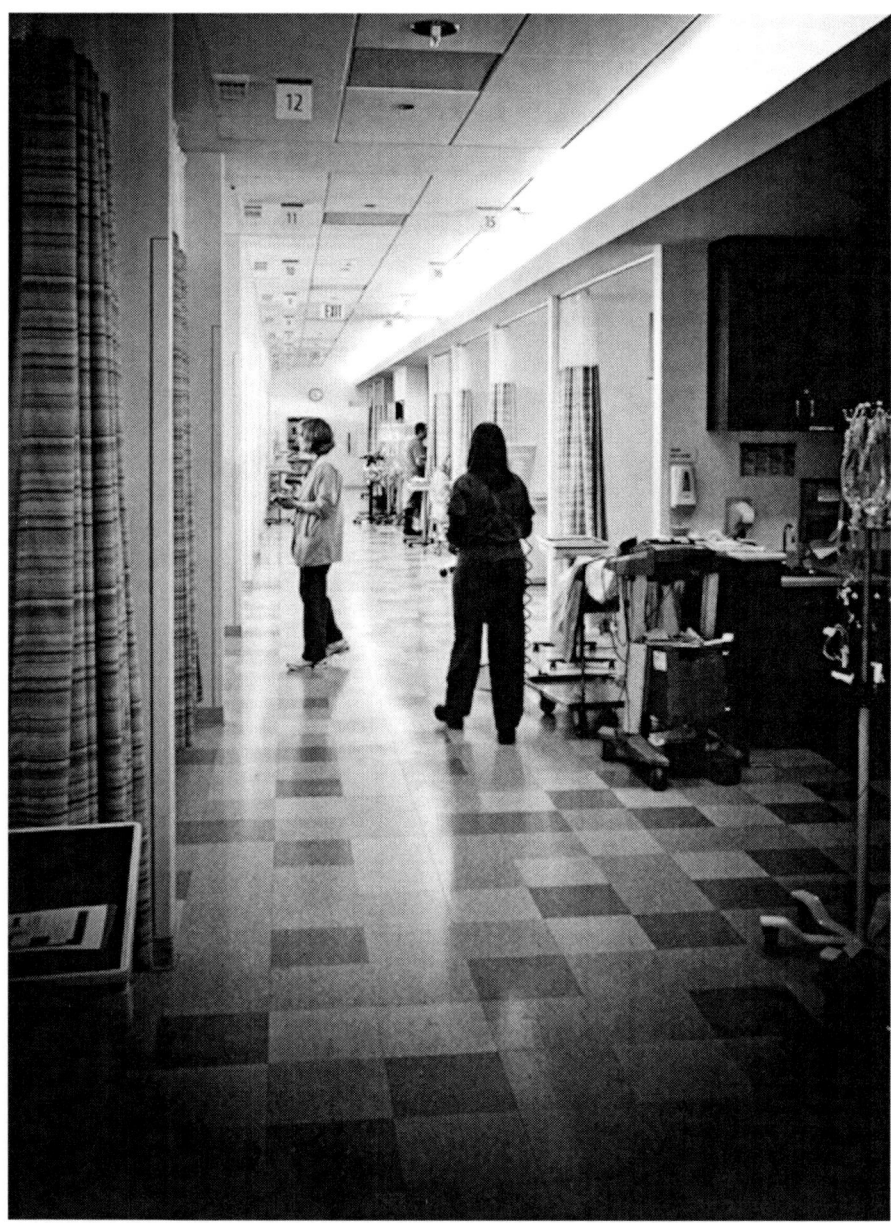

But first, we have more waiting before we go down another hallway like this one, to a surgery that no one should ever have to "consent" to, so we can come out the other side of hell and start a new life worthy of the heartbeats she is sacrificing so much for.

Final Approach

March 13, 2011

I am sure that there is a fatigue among the readers about all the whining I'm doing prior to surgery. Yeah, I have a problem with it (the surgery, not the fatigue), but that problem has painfully and slowly changed to an acceptance that this really needs to be done. Her meds only increase, and the benefits only last so long before she is back to suffering. No, if I really love her, I will escort her to this surgery with strength and confidence, and hide my fear and depression from her as long as I can. I'm not sure what good that does, she can read me like no other on earth. She knows my fear, she shares it. I only get to imagine her physical pain, but my imagination is very, very vivid right now.

Our tickets are punched. We will be together until they take her into surgery. At that point, she sacrifices body parts for future heartbeats and I wait. Strangers will cut out the cancer and I will have to trust and wait. When I finally see her in Intensive Care, she will be heavily sedated. She will be treated as well as strangers can treat her, but she is still a medical anomaly to them, an orthopedic / physiological / oncology problem to be solved with scalpels and sutures and skin grafts. I will not be able to touch her soul, see her eyes for days. She will be "sleeping" for up to a week, and I will be waiting, less alive, but waiting.

What was once theoretical and in the future, once measured in weeks is now measured in hours, and soon will be measured in minutes. I desperately want to throw the brakes on and pause everything, have more time to consider this, but the cancer does not wait, it does not lessen the pain while we consider our actions yet one more time. No, this is on schedule and it's going to happen to someone who truly does not deserve this. Even in the best of scenarios, the outcome is a soul that deserves all its freedom confined to a body compromised. I promise her with all my soul that her body will not become a dungeon. We will have a fuller life than we've ever known – damn the canes, crutches and wheelchairs.

And I promise her family that I will bring her home again. You will get to see her soul as alive as she's ever been, face to face.

I have spoken to all the surgeons. I have spoken to the insurance company. I have even made my final desperate pleas to God. Her body has defected to the enemy and now it's time to descend to yet another ring of hell to get back what can be saved. Regardless of her body, I assure you, her soul will be intact.

So our approach to all this is the same as it's been since we met — strength, courage and optimism about the future, tempered by moments of fear, doubt and sometimes outright panic.

We intend to cheat cancer one more time, but at a greater cost than previously ever imagined. We also intend to live a life better than we previously ever imagined.

If anyone can pull it off, it's us.

Stay tuned.

Surgery Day

March 16, 2011

Today is the first of two 12 hour surgeries for Carole. This morning, FOUR surgeons waited patiently in line at my wife's bedside for their turn to speak to her about their individual role over the course of today.

The plan includes cutting off all blood supply to the tumor. Finally we get to get back at the bastard.

And we did get some optimistic news. Our neurosurgeon flew all the way to Johns Hopkins to consult with other surgeons about the specifics of this case. What he told us is that if he can save the L5 nerve, she may be able to walk.

We won't know that until after Friday's surgery. Stay tuned...

The Walking Tour of Hell — Part 1

March 16, 2011

Yeah, I know I've used the word 'hell' to an abusive level lately, but the week of my wife's surgeries was the most intense ring of medicine and emotion that I can imagine experiencing. This ring is reserved for VIP's, not the typical tourists.
Lucky us.

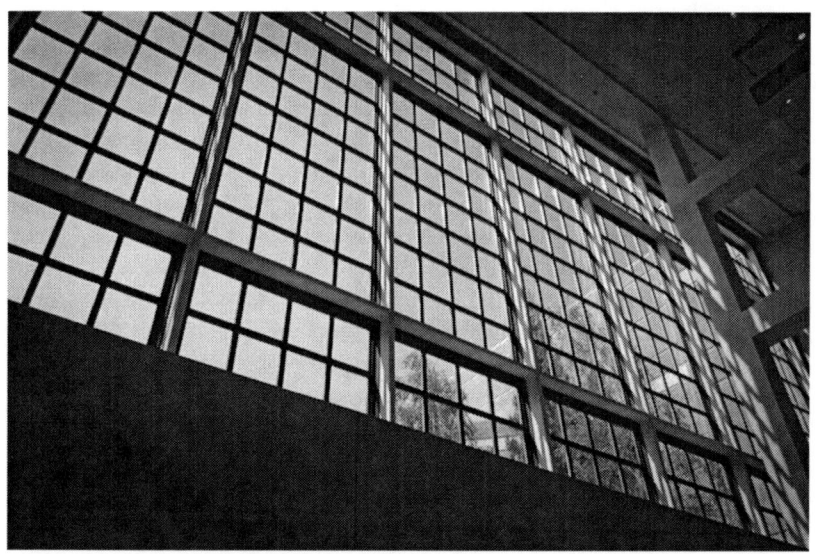

The day and night before the first surgery was filled with mental images I will never forget. Carole sitting at home, pausing, as if to gather her courage to get in the car and make the trek into a life-changing and perhaps tragic week; Carole weeping and shaking the night before surgery, asking what she had done to earn this fate. Carole consoling me as my tears fell unceasingly down my cheeks just before they took her away for this last-ditch attempt to save her life and end her suffering. No, there are no digital pictures of these moments that I can share, but these moments are all cataloged in my soul and will never leave me.

The surgical plan was to have two separate surgeries spread over three days. Wednesday was the 'setup' for Friday's surgery where the sacrum and the attached tumor would be removed in one piece, and the hole in my wife's lower back referred to as "the void" would be filled with replacement tissue. Each surgery was actually multiple "procedures". On a normal day, that "procedure" would be called a surgery. In our case, surgical teams would come and go, each with its own set of goals.

Typically, in pre-op it's a one-to-one ratio of surgeons to patients. In our case, Wednesday morning, there were four surgeons lined up to speak to Carole, each explaining their role in the "master plan" hatched by our neurosurgeon. And behind them were the residents, and behind them were the surgical nurses. We were rock stars that morning, everyone wanted a glimpse at "the patient" who was about to endure "the surgery" so risky and so rarely performed.

There is a lighted board in the pre-op area that tells the nurses which surgeon is working with which patient. In our case, there were four names that were responsible for the five "procedures" being done to one patient. Let me make this clear, these were five separate surgeries to be completed throughout the day. Twelve hours was the projected time table for all this activity, but everyone fully acknowledged that time was not a consideration; they would keep her on the table for as long as it took to get the setup for Friday completed.

In the midst of all this curiosity was our neurosurgeon, a young man who inspires confidence well beyond his years. Yeah, I know, every story needs a hero. This story has two, Carole and the neurosurgeon. His sole purpose was to free my wife from cancer and his strengths were caring, integrity and preparation. Not only did he fly to Johns Hopkins to meet with another surgeon about Carole's case, he actually practiced inserting the titanium rods that would make up my wife's lower back on a cadaver. I am a musician and I know the value of practice. He practiced the surgery over and over in spite of this being his TENTH surgery of this kind.

I don't know about you, but this is the kind of doctor I'd want in any situation. He refused to allow chance to play a part in this life-changing event and frankly, I want to be just like him when I grow up. Is he a hero? Hell yeah. There I go using "hell" again, but this man was committed body and soul to get my wife out of hell. The saying goes that fools go where angels fear to tread. This man is no fool, and he went where no one else was willing to go, including some Stanford doctors.

Again, I ask you, "Hero"? Again and again I answer, "Yes".

The typical beauty of Stanford Hospital closed around me like prison bars as I waited the twelve hours for the completion of Carole's first surgery.

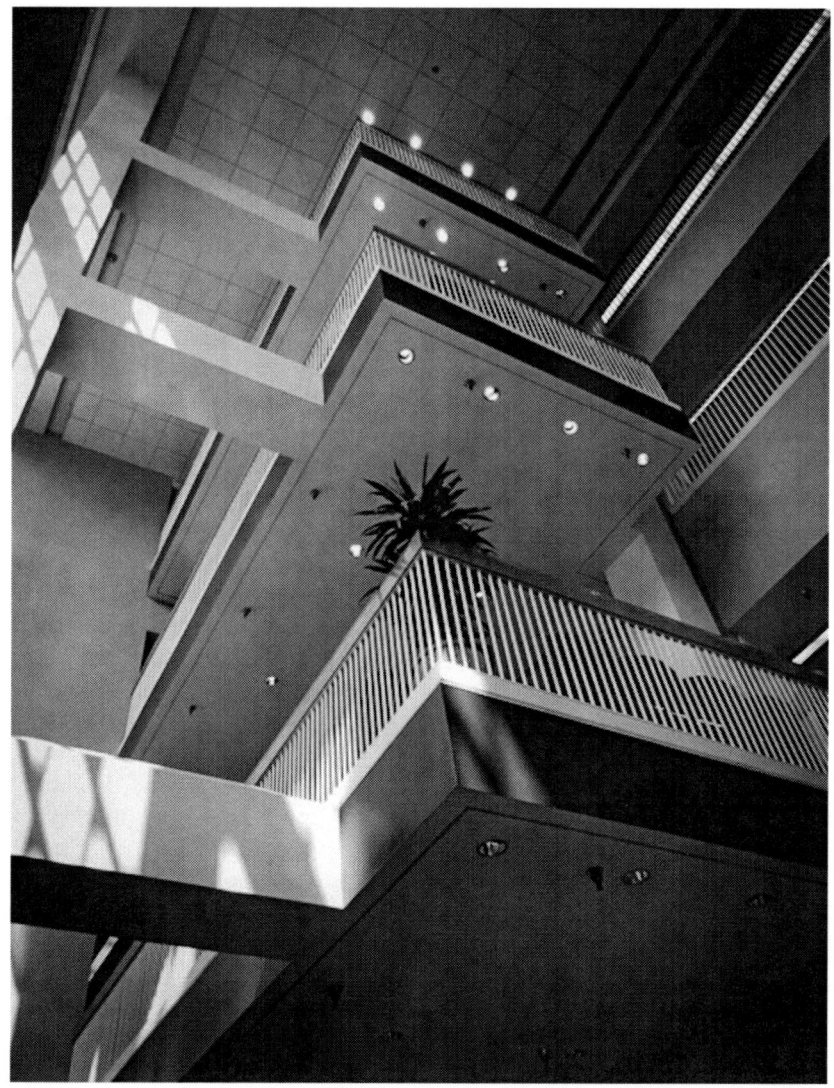

As each procedure ended, the surgeon responsible would come and speak to me. When the urology surgeon came out he enthusiastically announced that he had been able to save her bladder. Carole and I had been emotionally prepared by this same surgeon to sacrifice her bladder to cancer. According to him, he was able to cut around the tumor and reattach a shortened ureter to her bladder, thus saving some precious real estate for the plastic surgeon. I had no idea how important this would be in the near future.

You see, once the neurosurgeon removed the sacrum and the coccyx, there was going to be a hole, a "void", that needed to be filled with tissue and muscle to replace what once was my wife's lower back. The first choice of the plastic surgeons was to use half of the rectus abdominus. If you or someone you know is "in shape", you can see their abdominal "six pack". The plan was to use three of the six to fill the void in her lower back. How do they do that? The plastic surgeon cuts off the right-side three of the six pack, bags it, and pushes it into the abdominal cavity without cutting the veins and arteries that feed it, and closes the wound. If everything goes to plan, on Friday he pulls the living skin and tissue from the abdomen through the pelvis and attaches it where the lower back once was. The urologist, by working around the tumor, saved the preferred tissue for the plastic surgeon, instead of making him pull muscle up from the butt or down from the back. I jokingly said that we had just pulled an inside straight. He laughed and then said something I found to be prophetic. He said he didn't want the inside straight; he wanted the royal straight flush. At that moment I realized I had been hoping for my wife's survival and her pain to be under control. These doctors didn't feel that was acceptable, they wanted to give her every opportunity for the fullest and most meaningful life they could give her.

My optimism began to rise, and rightfully so. Every surgeon came out with the same message. 'It went perfectly'.

My optimism soared when the neurosurgeon came out and told me the L5 nerve was not involved with the tumor. It had been clear for a while that the S1 and S2 nerves in the sacrum would be sacrificed with the sacrum. It was not clear as to whether the L5 nerve was involved from the medical imagery. The L5 nerve allows you to pick up your foot, as when you tap your toes. The S1 allows you to push off your foot, as when pushing down on the gas pedal...or walking. (S2 controls bowel and bladder control).

So his statement could be paraphrased like this: with the L5 intact, some lengthy and painful physical therapy... and guts, my wife would not have to be wheelchair-bound for the rest of her life.

Yes, at that time the feeling I had was that prayers were being answered left and right, but a little voice inside me kept whispering that it's too early, there is too much time and too many things that need to be done for such optimism.

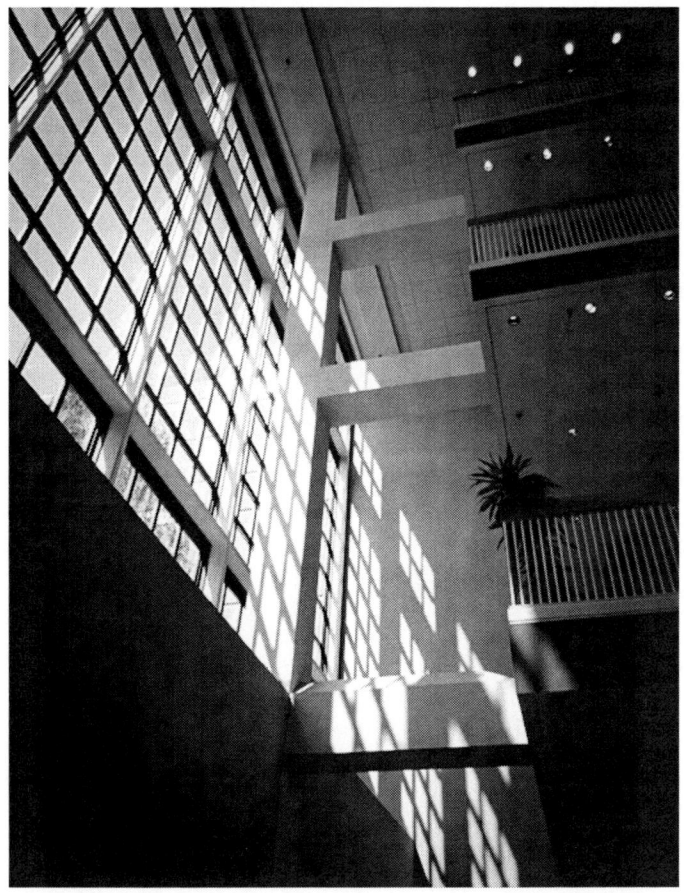

Day turned into night, and eventually I got to see my wife in the surgical intensive care unit. She had a breathing tube down her throat and would squeeze my hand to communicate with me. She was agitated from the tube and in considerable pain as the nursing staff tried to manage it, among other things. The mental image I have is of her flailing her arms weakly, almost as if the IV lines were too heavy for her to lift. Her eyes were semi open, but not focusing. She opened and closed her mouth trying to dislodge the breathing tube and trying to speak. Her skin was pale from blood loss and, to me at least, she was alive, but only at the most basic level.

I stood back to give the nurses the room they needed, but soon I was asked to leave. As I walked down the corridor from the ICU the optimism from earlier left me, like a balloon deflating, and I ended up literally dropping face first into a chair in the waiting room. My legs stopped working and all the lies I had been telling myself finally came to an end. I cried, I sobbed, I wept, I completely collapsed. No, I honestly cannot handle this. No, I honestly cannot help her. No, I honestly cannot get up anymore.

It was at that time that I felt two arms surround me in a bear-hug from behind. It was my friend Rick. He and his wife Denise insisted on coming to Stanford to sit with me for these days of surgery in spite of my protests. Rick's bear-hug was not intended to lift me; it was intended to share my every tear and every fear. It was intended to let me know I was not alone here. It was an offering of deepest compassion and strength. It was his way of saying that if my strength was gone, then take his.

And take I did. That same little voice that was warning me about optimism was now telling me to get up. It was telling me that I could not help anyone if I stayed this deflated. And it was also saying 'Jesus Christ, get up. If Carole saw you like this she would kick your ass.'

It's a wise little voice I have inside of me.

I got up, pulled myself together and we all left the hospital some 17 hours after I had pushed Carole through these same corridors in her wheelchair. With a day of surgeries completed, those hours were truly a lifetime ago. She could not physically go back to what she was in that wheelchair. The transformation had started and, as optimistic as the day was, it was still one damn tough day on everyone.

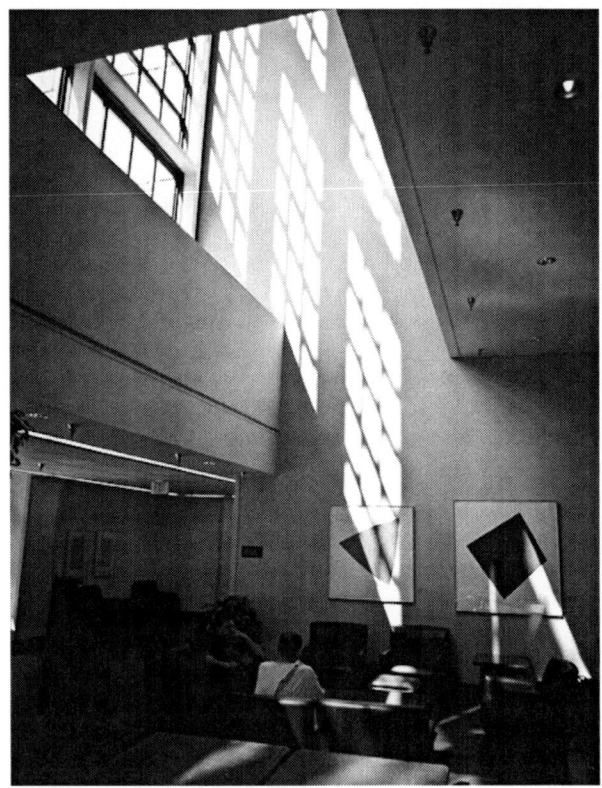

And we had three more days to go...

The Walking Tour of Hell — Part 2

March 18, 2011

Thursday was a silly, wasted day of optimism. Somehow, I was able to ignore the quiet conservative voice in my head that warned against such things. I saw Carole in the surgical ICU, and witnessed for myself how comfortable she was, how her pain was now "controlled", and how her struggling stopped once the breathing tube was removed. We had been warned by one resident that there was a high likelihood that my wife would be asleep for the day between surgeries but she here she was — awake, talking and making sense. The staff in the ICU was very impressed with how she was responding, and all of them stated that to me at every opportunity.

Between ICU visiting hours I went to the hospital gift shop and bought a deck of cards. I had come up with an idea for a picture using the playing card reference that one of the surgeons had given me, and Rick helped me brainstorm and shoot pix throughout the hospital.

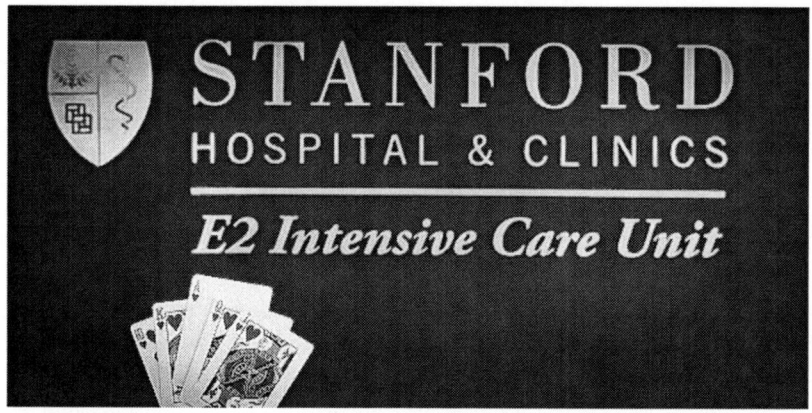

I decided that the royal straight flush should be in hearts since it showed my love for my wife and God's love for us. I mean, come on, we were batting one thousand through procedure after procedure. Surely, we were 'blessed', surely this was going to go as perfectly as Wednesday had. Faith can sometimes carry you and sometime blind you, both figuratively and literally.

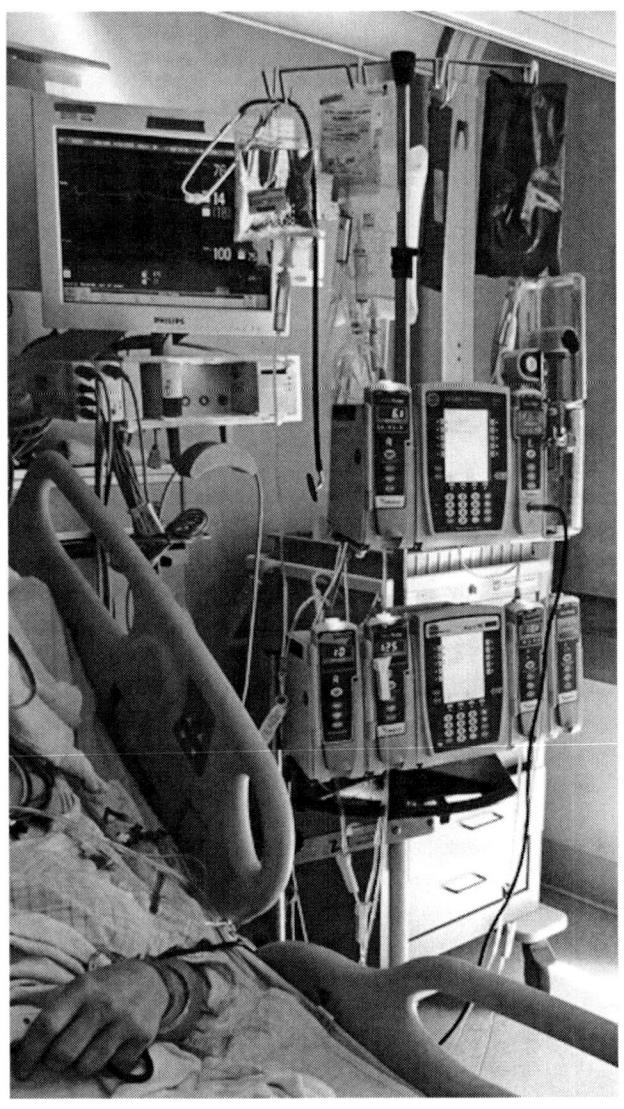

I took a picture of the various IVs that were running into my wife, since collectively they reminded me of R2D2, but the quiet voice in my head was getting louder by the heartbeat. Between shoots and conversations, Rick and I both spent quiet time with Carole. She was exhausted but she liked hearing the sound of our voices in her room.

All this good news and optimism only made Friday's surgery more valuable, more critical. Almost everything from Wednesday's surgeries could be reversed if needed. Friday's surgery had no such room for error. If there is an "all in" moment in a person's life, this was Carole's. All the "setup" would be wasted effort with one mistake, one unforeseen complication on Friday. Optimism has no value at a time like this, only reality, and the reality was sinking in savagely. Friday's surgery was not just important, but profoundly important in my wife's life.

This thought ground on me all afternoon and all night. I slept very little Thursday night into Friday morning. I had asked for a 3:30 am wake up call. I was awake well before that, and I think I woke the front desk person when I called to cancel the wake up call.

I hit the showers, found a Diet Coke and made my way to the hospital by 4:45 am. When I peeked in on Carole, her room was dark and she was napping. I did not disturb her. I made my way to the waiting room and sat in solitude for the hospital to wake up around me.

By 5:30 am she was awake and being prepped for surgery. I stayed with her until 7:30, when they finally rolled her from ICU to surgery. I went as far as I could, gave her a kiss, and then lumbered back to the waiting area for the duration. I can honestly tell you that any optimism from Thursday had been completely drained from me and replaced with concern. And not the typical "I hope she'll be all right" concern, but the heavy, crushing concern of believing everything the doctors say, except for everything the doctors say. My belief in everything was being challenged.

I would have given my soul at that moment to be in the operating room with her, to be the one responsible for saving every iota of quality of life that I could for her. I felt empty and helpless watching families slowly migrate through the waiting area as their loved ones went through similar, but less risky surgeries that morning.

I was reminded of game show contestants again. Some families were clearly winners; their loved ones had been spared from a dark prognosis by the skill of the Stanford surgeons. Others were not so lucky. Families literally collapsed onto one another as the surgeon gave them the news that the prognosis was dark or even darker still. Some families kept vigils up until the end, some families left immediately with no such vigil to attend to. The waiting room that day had been transformed into a threshold between worlds that it never became on Wednesday. Today, trust and guarantees were earned, not given. Today, the bus to the next life was running and not hurting for passengers. Today, the coin of the realm was concern, and I was a very, very rich man.

If you ever find yourself in a similar place, you will notice that time changes. It does not move at the same pace as any other day in your life. Each minute carries a cost and a burden that you have no choice but to pay and lift. And in the words of my brother-in-law, they are very heavy lifts.

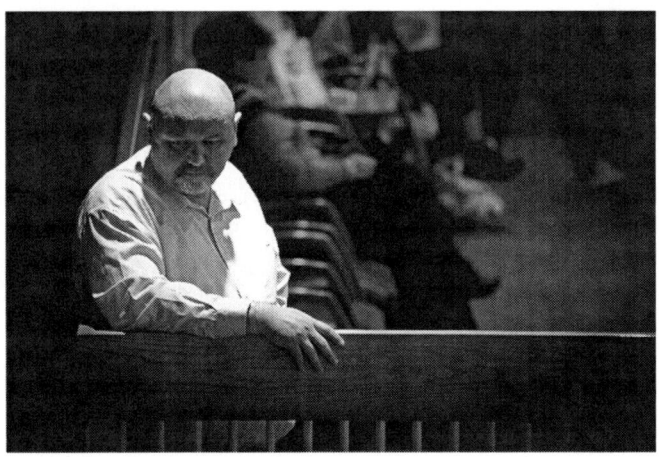

Picture by Rick Horowitz www.soshootme.com

Let me try to explain what waiting was like. Imagine that each minute was separated by a pane of glass. Over those sixty seconds a pressure builds within you from impatience, desperation and a kind of insanity. This pressure finally shatters the glass between this minute and the next, only to build up again. This is repeated sixty times an hour, for as many hours as it takes. You soon leave exhaustion well behind and venture into a physical and mental state that my language has no word for. It's a semi-controlled insanity that often drifts into insanity itself.

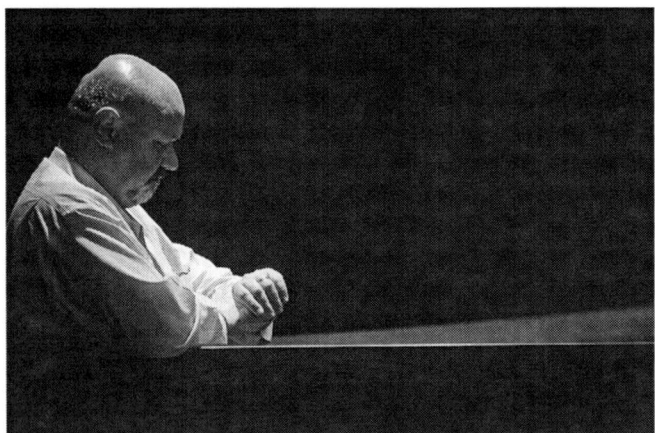

Picture by Rick Horowitz www.soshootme.com

I was often asked by Rick or Denise if I was "all right". No my dear friends, I was never "all right", I was at a precipice between faith and pure emotional collapse. The wind could have easily blown me in either direction. Checking my watch became a rote exercise, muscle memory kicked in when I wasn't even thinking about checking the time. Panes of glass dividing the minutes had become mounds of painful shards at my feet. A step in any direction just served to remind me of another wasted minute, another set of wasted breaths and heartbeats.

After waiting since 4:45 am, the neurosurgeon met us at about 9:45 pm. Everything went very well he said. He said that the tumor was bigger than expected, some three of his fists wide. He said she was being worked on by the plastic surgeon now and we could expect to see her in 45 minutes.

The next 45 minutes were even more difficult, as if the panes of glass between minutes had doubled in thickness, but they eventually passed.

I was warned by the anesthesiologist that my wife's face would be grossly swollen from surgery. You see, her hips were elevated for back surgery, elevated higher than her feet and head, and the natural body fluids would pool in her face and neck. When I finally saw her I was not prepared to see an unfamiliar face, one so swollen that it challenged me to identify her. Her face was easily twice its normal size and even her very eyeballs were protruding like they didn't belong to her face anymore.

I was assured by the medical professionals who surrounded me that all of this would return to normal as the fluids drained. I found myself as challenged to stay strong as I had been Wednesday evening, but this time I managed to hold together.

Partly from exhaustion, partly from fear, I left my wife in the care of the nurses who so brilliantly pulled her together previously, and headed back to my small rented room.

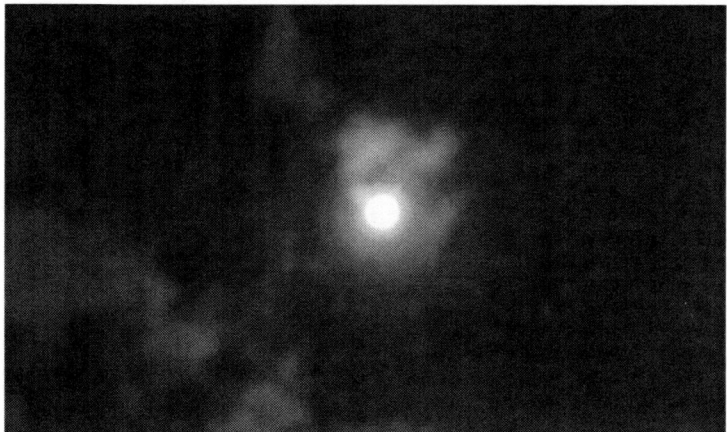

Once away from the hospital, I started to regain my optimism. "This wasn't so bad," I thought, "the neurosurgeon told us that everything went perfectly."

As I parked my car and headed to my room, I was struck by the "super-moon" that had parted the stormy skies above me. Most new beginnings start with a sunrise, our new beginning began with a bright full moon piercing the darkness, an apt symbol for the struggle we had been through.

My optimism lulled me to sleep that night, and woke me the next morning, but, as always, reality was just a step away.

Intermission

I have to interrupt the timeline here.

Carole's surgeries were on a Wednesday and a Friday. I stayed with her at Stanford until late Sunday, before I had to drive back home for work on Monday. I worked a short week and returned to her as soon as I could. I needed to maintain a minimum number of hours to keep my health insurance since I had already burned through vacation and sick time. This continued until she was transferred to a 'skilled nursing' facility in town.

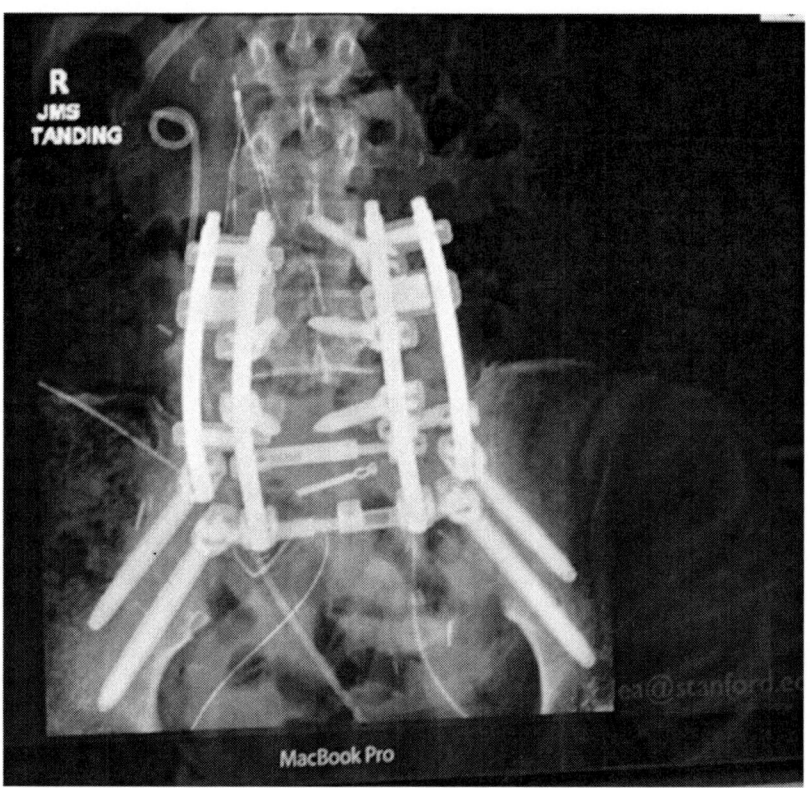

Carole's X-Ray as viewed from Dr. Mindea's computer.

Also, on the day after Carole's second surgery (March 19, 2011), the neurosurgeon called me and asked to meet with me in the cafeteria. He had tears in his eyes when he told me that, even with all the precautions in place, blood flow to Carole's eyes had been compromised sometime during the seventeen hours of surgery.

He had called Ophthalmology in and they examined her. The prognosis was not good. Her left eye was completely gone, and her right eye was significantly impaired. There was hope that *some* of the vision could return over time, but it was doubtful that it would change dramatically.

This is information that I chose to keep from family and friends for the time being. First, I needed to process it and discuss it with Carole, and second, family and friends had been through enough. They needed a break as badly as I did. This could keep, especially if it was permanent.

On top of all this, and unbeknownst to me, Carole's post-surgical blood test showed a large amount of an enzyme that indicated heart trouble during surgery. We both found out much later that cardiology's term for this was "moderate size heart attack."

The writing from this point on is chronologically honest and, in places, innocently optimistic.

Another "M" Word

March 26, 2011

I have to interrupt this pity party blog series with some breaking news.

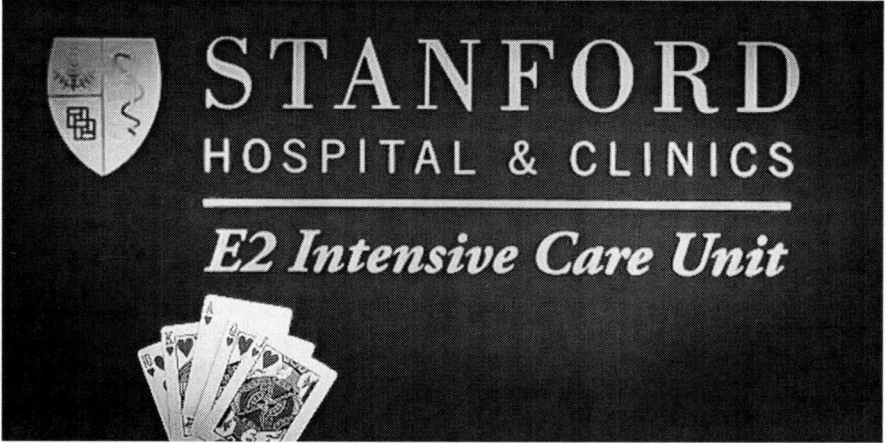

I can be an idiot sometimes. That's not the news, but it is important background information, keep it in mind.

I walked into Carole's room in the ICU this morning just as she was starting her exercises. The Physical Therapy and Occupational Therapy staff had given her some simple exercises to do while lying in bed. She does stuff like make punching motions in the air, raise her legs and wiggle her feet.

It was during the feet wiggle portion that I noticed that she could move her feet both up AND down. I watched silently as she went through the entire series of motions for three complete sets.

During each set I watched her point her toes up to the head of the bed, as I expected her to be able to do, and then down to the foot of the bed. "What an idiot I am," I thought, "You told everyone that once the S1 nerve was cut, she would not be able to point her foot. You're going to have to go tell everyone that you misunderstood the neurosurgeon and confess your idiocy to family and friends," (Yes, I confess I was in a good mood this morning because I was with Carole again and now I could actually help her instead of just talking to her on the phone).

After she was done, I held her feet and asked her to point her toes towards the head of the bed while I provided some resistance. She did it with no problem, except that her left foot was weaker than her right. That made sense since she had been favoring her left foot and leg since the tumor made its appearance. I hoped, and still hope that this is a case of muscle atrophy and not permanent weakness.

I then asked her to point her toes to the bottom of the bed, as if she were pushing down on two gas pedals. Her right foot was so strong that I was surprised, so much so that I told her she could drive with that foot just the way it was. Her left foot was lacking but again, I chalked this up to atrophy.

After lunch I got a call from the neurosurgeon on my cell phone. He was at Carole's bedside and wanted me to join him. I ran up to the third floor from the cafeteria and got to shake his hand and say thanks (again). I told him that in my non-medical opinion, Carole was looking and doing great. He reassured me that my diagnosis of the patient was correct. We followed that up with a conversation about how long Carole would be staying and where she might be discharged to.

Just as we were finishing up, I remembered to ask that question from this morning. The conversation went something like this:

Me: "Hey Doc, I must have misunderstood something. I thought Carole would not be able to point her toes after the S1 nerve was cut. I noticed this morning that she could do that."

Intelligent, compassionate Doc: "Yeah, I saw that, too. So did my two residents."

Me: "So how come she can do that?"

Intelligent, compassionate Doc: "I honestly don't know."

I immediately rewound the little tape machine in my head and listened to his answer again. Not satisfied with the aural quality of the recording I blurted out "You don't know?"

Intelligent, compassionate Doc: "That's right. I wish I knew the answer why, it's embarrassing as the attending neurosurgeon not to be able to answer a question from my residents."

Not a flock, but a fleet of butterflies were released in my stomach. It's a big stomach, but it still got very crowded.

Me, in an almost whispered voice: "Are you serious?"

Intelligent, compassionate Doc: "I can attest to you that I cut both S1 nerves and I still don't know why she can do that."

I turned and asked my wife to do it again, not only to confirm her physical abilities but my sanity as well. She did, but she was obviously bored with the whole thing.

I moved up to the head of the bed so I could see my wife face to face and said to her "Carole, you're going to walk again. You're going to walk again!"

She was tired and not sharing my excitement so I turned to the neurosurgeon. He just stood there with a little smile and his hands in his lab coat pockets. He didn't dispute me, but he didn't agree. Surgeons can only speak about sure things, not possibilities in a case like this. But the silence was golden to my ears.

After he left, I replayed the conversation in my head multiple times and annoyed my wife by asking her to do the "lead foot" exercise one more time.

It is now 8:30 pm, and I am stunned and scared by this news. I know this post is written in a light-hearted way, but now I am as serious as I can get when I say that this is not planned, this is not a way to create drama or gain attention. I am as serious as my own heart attack, she can move her feet in a way we were told she would not be able to.

I called one friend who is in the religion business, and his explanation was simple — it was a miracle. I called another friend who is in the medical business who was reluctant to jump on the miracle bandwagon just yet. Hers is a world of scientific proof, but she had no explanation, just like our Stanford neurosurgeon. Right now, the miracle band is playing WAY louder than the scientific band as bands on bandwagons go.

So, miracle or medicine?

Look, right now I feel like an idiot. Here I was begging and pleading for a miracle, and now that I get it, I am reluctant to believe it. I asked God thousands of times in hundreds of ways for a treatment, or a cure, or some way to remove the tumor and still leave her walking, and here one lands in our lap and I don't believe it.

With loyalty and fidelity like that, if you were God right now, why wouldn't you just pull the plug and start over? (If you're looking for a more eloquent way to put this, see Psalm 144).

I am such an idiot, such a human idiot, too scared to believe, and too scared not to believe.

What a freaking hero. What a weak fool.

Now my one prayer, the one most sincere prayer of my life after a week of sincere prayer, is this:

Please let this miracle be permanent.

The picture at the top of this post now has far more meaning than I ever dared to imagine.

Stairway to Heaven

March 31, 2011

Today has been a long time in coming.

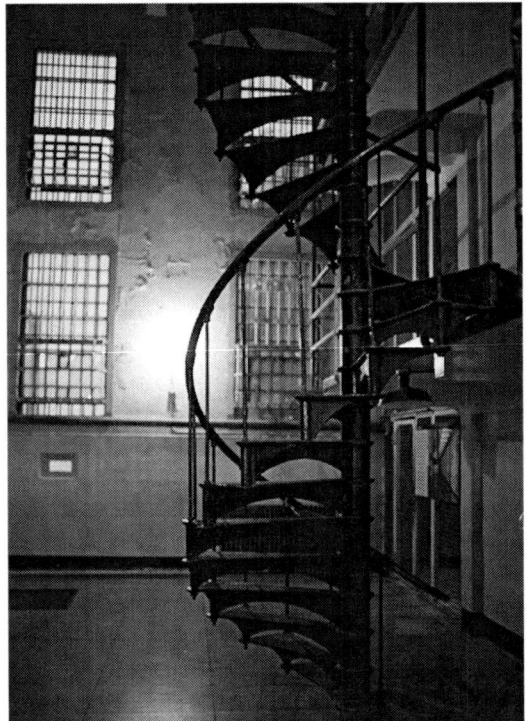

Today, I can attest that hell has a back door.

Today, my wife is being transferred from Stanford University Hospital to a skilled nursing facility in town. She will spend as much time as needed there, until she is strong enough to be transferred to a physical therapy facility. From there she goes home, and continues what might be a year of additional physical therapy.

It's not going to be easy, but it's pain for a purpose versus the useless pain of cancer.

It's a step-by-step journey out of the suffering she endured for so long, and any step out of hell is a step toward heaven, right?

Passing Through

March 31, 2011

Carole's new temporary home is deep in the heart of downtown Fresno. Like many downtowns across America, the glory days of this downtown are decades in the past. It's a neighborhood of older homes, some kept up and some run down. Across the street is a shelter for battered women and their children. It's a neighborhood littered with churches and chapels, most with a sign out front with an optimistic message such as "the truth shall set you free". Some of the people who live there have lived there all their lives, some not, but all of the people who live in this area now need optimism wherever they can find it because, economically speaking, their American Dream stopped here, left them off and they're not going anywhere else.

The residents in my wife's new temporary home cannot see these signs from their windows, and rightfully so, since, like their neighbors, regardless of "the truth", few of them will ever be set free.

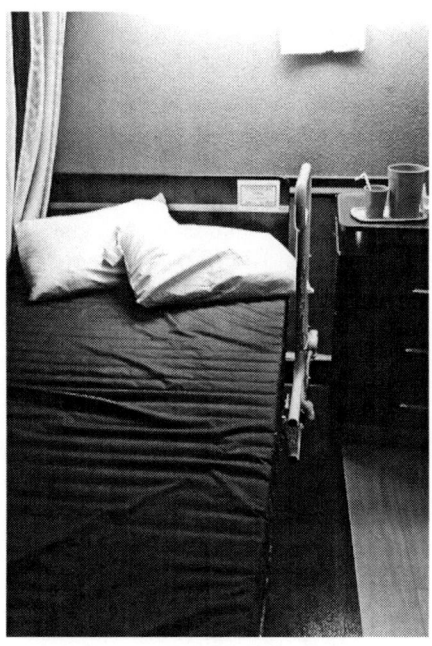

For the record, the last time I saw my wife was Sunday in a hospital some 160 miles away. That day there was no discussion of discharge from anyone. On Monday a rumor started about a discharge "soon". On Tuesday, it was "where do you want to move your wife to?" I took Tuesday afternoon off from work to look through the options my insurance company allowed me, and made some visits. Since it was not clear if we needed a "skilled nursing" or a "physical rehabilitation" facility, I had to visit both types in just a few hours.

The physical rehab facilities were state of the art and the thought of leaving my wife there was actually comforting to me. On the other hand, the skilled nursing facilities were depressing and downright scary.

I started with an "award winning" skilled nursing facility which was across town but hopefully worth the drive.

I was appalled. It was clean but small, creating the sense of overcrowding. As residents left their rooms they only added to the congestion in the halls. Walking in a straight line was a luxury reserved for third shift. The feeling in the place was not joy or hope, but busy, and not in a productive way. I imagined how difficult it must be to get a bandage changed or even a pain pill here. No, I decided I cannot leave my wife here, even for a few weeks. I could not imagine how someone could leave a family member here for the rest of their life.

A buddy of mine called places like this "warehouses". I completely understand his meaning now. My Dad used to call places like this "God's waiting room". I'm glad my Mom had enough respect for him to let him die at home.

I pray I will be shown the same courtesy.

In comparison to the 'award winner', the place my wife is at now was nirvana that afternoon. A new owner has taken over and the remodeling is in full swing. She will get physical therapy twice a day until she is strong enough to be transferred to a modern acute physical rehabilitation hospital. She is on the second of six floors which, luckily for us, is a remodeled floor.

Again, for the record, it's one thing to tour a facility under pressure, and completely something else to actually see your wife in their bed, on their floor.

She arrived about 7 pm and was alone in her room when I entered. She had been delivered there by paramedics and, until the point of my arrival; no one had spoken to her. She was thirsty and in pain from the drive, so I quickly left and introduced myself to the staff and got things moving. In twenty minutes she had water and pain meds. Soon after that I asked where the linens were kept and then proceeded to cool my wife down with a wet face cloth.

Once she started getting comfortable, I started to inspect the room. It was not "clean", but "clean enough". If not for the drone of the roof-mounted fan outside her window, she would have been deafened by the sound from televisions, all on different channels, coming from the hall. It was humid in her room, and I asked a staff member to turn on the air conditioning. She returned with a pair of fingernail clippers to turn on the AC, since the knob was missing. I'm not sure how much good it will do, since it's "against the rules" to close your door.

As the pain meds kicked in and my wife got drowsy, I started to notice the steady stream of residents walking past the door. They could not see Carole because I had pulled the privacy curtain, but they were still walking by, looking at me. It took me a while, but eventually I figured out that this new resident they were so curious about had a precious commodity, a visitor. One small, elderly lady kept passing by, asking with her eyes "Can you see me, am I still here, will you talk to me?" On one of my errands to the front desk, I made sure to ask her how she was doing. She reacted like a flower to water and sun. She stretched out to her whole five foot frame, blinked her eyes and smiled. In her finest lady-like posture she said 'I am fine, thank you for asking'. I was tempted to ask her to dance, right there in the hall. I wanted her to know that yes, I saw her and still recognized the lady she once was. I wanted to show her the respect that she once knew daily in this place of disrespect and where time stands still. But I was on a mission of comfort for my wife, and nothing comes before that. I hope our dance is only postponed.

Another elderly female resident called me a "mountain of a man" and asked if my father was in the bed. No I told her, my wife was in the bed. She seemed surprised, as if I had married a woman forty years my elder. She seemed to have difficulty comprehending that we were just passing through.

And that's precisely when the thought struck me. We were just passing through.

This place, like suffering from cancer, like being trapped in a wheelchair, like being trapped in unspeakable pain, like undergoing so many surgeries in such a short time and literally re-engineering a human body, was just a another step on our way up the ladder, away from the belly of hell and on our way to a place far closer to heaven than we've been in months. As guilty as I felt about leaving my wife in this place, I did take comfort in knowing that we would someday soon be leaving, unlike the residents surrounding us. Yes, our time might come where we find ourselves lowered again to this ring of hell, this ring that erases what you were, this ring that devalues your worth to the level of your physical abilities, this ring that abandons you to heartbeats you don't want, a useless life unimagined in your youth.

But not today.

We still have a tomorrow filled with physical therapy and physical pain, but with a hope of regaining much of what cancer stole, and much of what time still owes us.

Honestly, tonight I feel like such a shit for abandoning her in such a place, as I struggle to remind myself that we are just passing through.

And unlike the residents of this place, or even the neighborhood, she still has glory days ahead of her.

So help me God.

Lucky Dog

April 3, 2011

I believe in God, the Creator of heaven and earth.
I also believe that He's not nearly the asshole he's been made out to be.

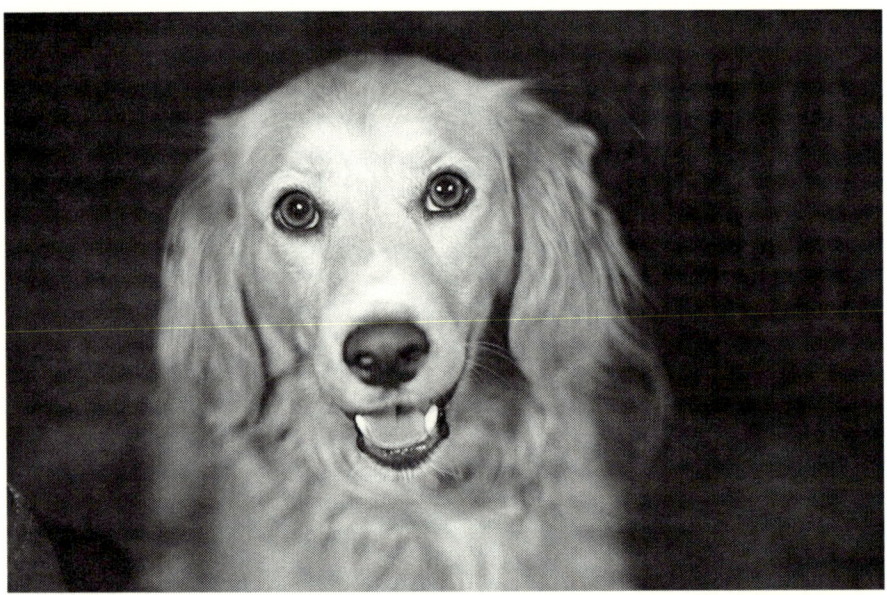

Let me let you in on a not-so-guarded secret. "Skilled nursing" is a code word for nursing home. Call it a retirement home, call it a rest home, call it a scrap heap of useless, used-up people, but the end result is the same. My wife is currently in a place where there is "skilled nursing" available 24/7, a place where she is supposed to be kept "comfortable", while awaiting physical therapy. (And by the way, is there such a place as "unskilled nursing"?)

In truth, as in all skilled nursing facilities, you hear things that disturb you. Some residents beg you to help them escape, some residents just sit and cry in their rooms for no apparent reason. And some, let's call them the "newbies", believe if you press the call button a nurse will come to your aid at her earliest convenience.

My wife has an advocate... me. If she is in need of anything, I lumber my fat ass down the hall to the nurse's station and ask a very specific person for very specific help for one very specific patient. The results I get are excellent, almost as if the staff respects a patient who has an advocate, as if this patient is not one of the 'forgotten' ones, forgotten by family and friends who inhabit most of the beds on the floor. No, the staff responds to flesh and blood requests, especially when they sense that this flesh and blood could morph into Tony Soprano in a New Jersey heartbeat. Ah yes, my East Coast roots still serve me well...

While running an errand for my wife (she wanted a cold can of iced tea from the vending machine) I met the most diminutive, white haired lady I have seen so far in the facility. I'm not sure if wheelchairs make people look that small, or if people really were that small once-upon-a-time, but she was waiting for the elevator to the first floor as I approached. Once the door opened, she could not navigate her way through the large containers they use to deliver meals to get on the elevator. I try to be more than just a pretty face in this world, and I managed to hold the elevator with one foot while pushing the containers aside so she could share my elevator to the first floor.

During the ride she told me she was heading to the vending machine to get a Snickers bar. I told her I was getting a can of iced tea for my wife, so maybe we could go together. What happened next was so cute that I almost cried.

I told her if she picked up her tiny feet that I would be glad to push her to candy-heaven. She was so surprised that someone would consider doing that for her, but up her tiny little feet went, and "zoom" we went down the hall. I was walking at slower-than-my-normal pace, but she was so happy that she didn't have to roll herself halfway down the length of the building for her treat.

We zigged and zagged around obstacles and people, and unwittingly, I "zoomed" her right past the vending machines in the common area. Before she could protest, I had zigged and zagged her into the old wing and down the long hall. You see, the staff had let me in on a secret a few nights ago. The vending machines with the coldest drinks and the most candy were in the staff break room on the first floor. Once I heard that, I never even looked for another place of refreshment.

My partner, who had just become my passenger, had no idea where we were headed, just that wherever we were going, we were going in one hell of a hurry compared to her natural pace.

I didn't exactly burn rubber on the turns, but I did emphasize the fun we were having by making engine noises all the way.

When I opened the door to the staff break room I heard her take in her breath, like we just found the Holy Grail. "Where are we?" she asked. "The staff break room," I answered. "I've never been here," she whispered. I never did ask her how long she had lived here, but I got the impression it was much longer than she deserved.

As I pushed her forward, she did an immediate inventory of all the candy bars that are just not available on other floors. She pointed at a candy bar and said, "That one!" and placed coins in my hand.

She said it was 90 cents for that candy bar. I checked the price and it was a dollar. I then checked my hand, and in it were eight dimes and a penny.

My math sucks, but I knew that my new, nameless friend was not leaving without her candy bar so I went to plan 'B'.

"Dear"', I said, 'it would be my privilege to buy a girl with such a sweet smile a candy bar tonight," At first she refused, but I was able to convince her that her money was no good in the staff break room, and that she would only make me happy by letting me buy her a rare and precious treat.

I got her the candy bar, and my wife the iced tea, and then we proceeded back to the elevator, but at a much slower pace. I didn't want to spoil the feeling that someone noticed her, that someone found her special. Once on the second floor she tried to give me her coins one more time, but I told her that her smile was all the reward I would ever need. Then I headed for my wife's room.

In truth, it was my pleasure. In truth, it was my privilege, and still is.

When I returned to my wife, I saw that her pain had taken a turn for the worse. Since leaving Stanford, her pain management had been a roller coaster, and was my number one job. Nurses cannot give drugs which doctors do not order, but at my request shift after shift of nurses had been calling doctors asking permission to increase the pain meds to a more effective level. I try to be as polite as I can, but the intensity of my request often catches the nurses off-guard. Honestly, I have seen enough of my wife's suffering for ten lifetimes. Enough is enough.

Every shift I introduce myself to the staff nurses, and ask for their help in stemming my wife's pain. They all feel badly, they all say the same caring things, but only one nurse truly understood.

I'll call her "Blue". As I started into my introduction and my request for timely pain management, I saw a look cross her face. It was a look of knowledge and of mourning and emotional pain.

I did not say a word, but Blue volunteered that she lost her husband last year, that the worst part for her was letting him go, but she knew he was no longer in pain, and how horrible the pain had become, especially at the end. She promised me that she knew what to do, and more importantly, she would do it.

I confess that of all the 'pain' I have endured (it's hard for me to use the word pain after seeing what my wife has been through), the most difficult pain recently is leaving her behind in the care of strangers. It's clear that all of the strangers know what to say, but few know the pain first hand, and know what to do.

I admit, after all the shift change meetings I made sure to attend, of all the staff members I met and tried to befriend, Blue was the first and only one who knew what the caregiver's hell is like. This was exactly the right person at exactly the right time.

Thank God.

And that leads me back to my creed at the top of this post.

God gets blamed for pain, and for cancer, and for suffering that was never his intention. Nowhere do you find mention of Adam needing narcotics to relieve the physical pain from his tumor, or Eve being put away for violating the sacred formula, the formula that says if you require more attention from your family than they can comfortably give, you end your life in 'skilled nursing', and very much alone.

God seldom gets credit for the little things, like a fat bald man making someone lonely feel special, or a still-grieving nursing professional helping relieve the concern of one very frustrated and concerned spouse.

I can leave her with a much greater sense of peace knowing that my pain resonates in 'Blue'. She will treat my wife tonight as she wished she could still treat her husband.

Her sadness becomes my peace.

Cancer is Lucifer's curse, it can't come from anywhere else, but the compassion that rises from that pain is a gift from a God that puts exactly what you need where you need it, when you need it.

God, the Creator of heaven and earth, gets a bad rap for "allowing" this to happen. Perhaps it's time to give credit where credit is honestly due. Lucifer is the asshole, so why is it so easy to believe in a God that allows suffering instead of the cold, selfish heart that enjoys suffering, abandonment and pain?

The picture at the top of this post is 'Reggie', Carole's favorite dog, whose picture hangs in Carole's room, reminding her of the unconditional love that awaits her when she finally returns home.

Reggie is unaware of Lucifer or his curses.

Lucky dog.

It's Nothing to Worry About, It's Only Pain.

April 4, 2011

I am exhausted.

Not in a physical way, but a deeply emotional way, the kind of exhaustion that only comes from marathons of pain and pain and pain. And it's not my pain, it's my wife's. I can not even express the frustration I feel while fighting to control her physical pain yet again. This is a special ring of hell reserved for spouses, and I've spent my allotted time here. My immediate urge is to inflict similar pain on someone responsible, so they can clearly understand how slowly time marches when you're hurting that badly. People who know me, know that this is never my first option, but it has become my preferred option, even though I cannot use it. Making another person suffer would be criminal, except for the medical professionals who "know better". I don't have a degree, so I cannot legally inflict pain on an innocent person without going to jail.

They can.

What a country.

I am my wife's advocate, a role I gladly take on, but it's a hard role to fulfill when the people you expect to help just ignore her as person or a patient.

I had to have a series of come-to-Jesus phone calls with the director of nursing at the facility my wife is currently a resident of. Why do I, a freaking idiot layman, have to tell the director of nursing, presumably an RN, that my wife having to wait twenty-four hours for a pain medication is unacceptable?

I honestly don't give a rat's ass where you get it from, just get it. And don't tell me you had it in a syringe in the 'emergency' kit this whole time and didn't use it because the doctor prescribed the same med in pill form.

These are the people I give my wife's life to while I have to work, or sleep. These are the people too busy to help her when she pushed the nurse call button to ask for pain meds. These are the people who sent a CNA trainee in to do a nurse's job. These are the people I went to visit today with a message that could not be misunderstood.

From now on, when my wife suffers, you suffer.

I am done talking to you. This is not baseball where you get three strikes, this is medicine and you're lucky to get one.

My next call, if needed, goes to my insurance company. I will tell them that all the money they spent on this dramatic surgery is going to waste because a certain "skilled" nursing facility in Fresno is holding up my wife's recuperation and therapy, because no one will answer the fucking nurse call button with a pill that is as common as aspirin in any pharmacy in America. I will ask my insurance company where they want me to move her, because the attention she is not getting is not worth the dollars the insurance company so carefully counts. I will tell them that I have entered my wife's room too often and witnessed her crying in her bed because no one will check up on her; no one will spend the five minutes to ease her pain.

I will tell the insurance company that they are paying for a hand job, a complete lie, if my wife spends more than a New Jersey minute in suffering again.

I wasn't born here, and where I come from, justice is not always served by judges and juries.

I sincerely and deeply regret that I cannot throw one punch in all this, but I will make sure the care for my wife, and all patients, in this facility gets better, or I will hit them in the only place they are capable of feeling pain; **their precious bottom line.**

I will speed dial your ass into having to explain yourself to the insurance company faster than you can say 'Press your call button'.

Try me.

It's nothing to worry about, it's only pain.

Good News, Bad News

April 5, 2011

The short story is this: the staff at the facility has a new attitude, brought about by an inspiring motivational address by the director of nursing.

The shorter story is this: good news travels fast, bad news travels faster.

The time from Carole pressing her call button to a response is now measured in a very small number of minutes, think single digits. There are still issues addressing her pain completely, but it's not from lack of attention as in previous nights.

And now that the pain meds are coming as scheduled, I am starting to see the pre-cancer Carole again, the woman with the dancing blue, mischievous eyes, the woman of quick wit and faster smirk.

This is the woman I promised my life to, and she is still in there. That's all the encouragement I need.

It's too early to tell the world that she's back, but it's not too early to announce she never left.

She'll be back, and on her own two feet, on her own terms, with no self pity or sorrow.

Because that's the way she wants it.

And so do I.

And reinforcements are on the way...

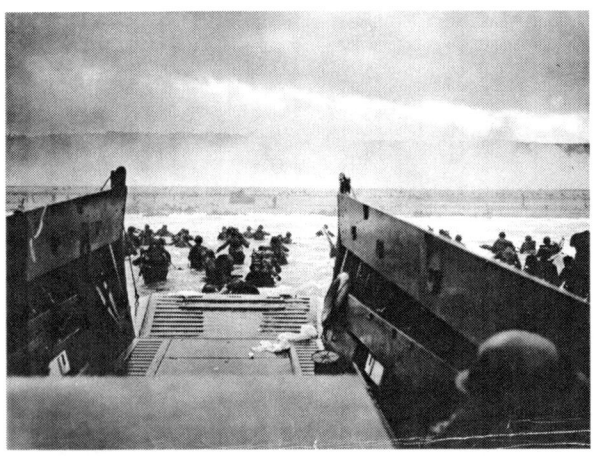

...Carole's Mom arrives again on Thursday. God help the world.

Tough News

April 11, 2011

As a concerned caregiver, I can tell you that my wife is getting stronger and, while there are good days and bad days, she is trending towards strength and healing.

Selfishly, I have to report my status as well.

My status is empty, emptier and emptiest. Watching your spouse suffer takes its own pound of flesh, but forging a team of strangers, even strangers in the medical field, is frustrating, difficult work, and sometimes impossible work. Strangers with medical training are still strangers, and only they can *decide* to care.

I have done my best to recruit and include the facility staff. I learn their names, tell our story to them, and try to make them a part of the solution. I even show everyone who has the stomach for it pictures of the post-surgical tumor. Some are impressed, some grossed out, but no one walks away untouched by the toughness shown by the lady in 203 B.

And tough she is. She is missing body parts that typically redefine a person's life into a list of limitations, but she is adjusting and making us believe that life, her *previous* life, will go on. Regardless of family, friends, or the completely clueless, the lady in 203 B is passing through, eventually leaving "skilled nursing"' behind on her own power, because of a higher power, and a stubborn streak that serves her well.

This woman, this lady, will eventually walk out where so many are wheeled out. She will put one foot in front of the other until she arrives home, into the love of her pets and the arms of those that love her.

She is tough, she is stubborn, and she will walk where others have only dreamed.

Patience will reveal everything.

Stay tuned.

Pass the Matches

April 12, 2011

I will try desperately not to turn this post into a whiney-gram, but I would like to share with you some of the sources of stress that a caregiver runs up against.

I walked into my wife's skilled nursing facility this week only to be met at the elevator by Mom-In-Law. The message was short and clear, your wife is in considerable pain and I cannot find a nurse anywhere. A quick recon of the second floor confirmed my Mom-In-Law's observation and a quick interrogation of the baby-faced nursing assistants told me that ALL the nurses in the building were in a meeting.

I rumbled like an angry tank to the Administrator's office and told her that my wife was in pain and I could not find a nurse on her floor. She echoed what I already knew, that they were all in a meeting. I raised my voice, and my intensity, considerably, "I don't care!" I am still not sure if my voice echoed throughout the building or the entire neighborhood, but it did through the administrator. For a full five seconds she just stared at me until she turned and said over her shoulder that she would call them now.

The elevators in this facility are very slow, so slow in fact that the nurses' meeting broke up and I rode up to the second floor with them. I smiled and kept a polite demeanor until the second floor crew and I spilled out of the crowded car. Once the door closed I informed the nurses that my wife had been pressing her nurse call button for 45 minutes and needed pain meds NOW.

To their credit, my wife had her meds in less than two minutes, and only had to wait an additional thirty minutes for them to kick in. For the luckily uninformed, pain is best managed BEFORE it starts. Once it starts to crescendo, it is a marathon measured in hours to get back under control. We have run this marathon much too often in the last few months. In fact, we have run it enough for both our lifetimes. This is the one single responsibility that I am exhausted from. Of all the things that medical professionals deal with, why is my wife's pain so insignificant?

Add to this stress the joy of trying to get a pair of glasses to replace my wife's newly broken frames without a prescription, and no, the not-very-helpful-eyeglass-lady was not helpful at all, even though the optometrist who wrote the expired prescription was in the same building. No, don't throw me clues, it's way more fun arguing with you for an hour. And thank you Miss not-very-helpful-eyeglass-lady for taking two hours to provide my wife's glasses in spite of the one hour service promise painted on the window.

Or how about trying to coordinate all of the follow up appointments from Stanford? Don't get me wrong, I love those guys and gals, but they don't realize that we are 160 plus miles away and we currently need medical transport to move Carole out of bed, forget about town. She cannot endure it, I will not allow it.

And I'm trying to work my full time job to keep my insurance and my part-time job for money, and my other part-time job (when they call) to keep the title of 'photographer', as selfish as that sounds.

If anyone asked me how I truly felt and honestly wanted to know the answer, I would tell them that I am in a barren, dry place, like Death Valley or the Bonneville Salt Flats. I would tell them that everywhere I turn the hot wind is blowing in my face and that the sun is cooking me where I stand. I would tell them that I am down on one knee, my muscles melting off my bones. On my right shoulder is another Earth. I am Atlas, holding one world from touching the world at my feet. I am being crushed, but there is no other place I belong.

My brother-in-law would call this a heavy lift. I disagree with every fiber I have left. This is a lift of a lifetime, worthy of the soul of a lifetime, hers.

No one will ever look at me and think "weight-lifter", or even "strength", like they do when they see my brother-in-law, but I don't need that. Just look at my wife when she defies the odds and walks into any room and think strength, determination, guts. Just think about her sacrifice, her refusal to bow to cancer, her ability to rise above near-impossible odds.

I am content to fall away into the echo of my wife's success. My purpose is served when she rises from the ashes. I kept my promise, and that is all I need to know to live a full life.

Her fire can be my ashes, as long as her Phoenix rises to its potential.

Pass the matches.

A Matter of Time

April 13, 2011

We know a very brave young woman who was diagnosed with breast cancer about the same time that Carole started her own cancer journey last fall. This beautiful young mother of two daughters endured a double mastectomy and is currently enduring the last of her chemo treatments.

Tomorrow morning, she is going to sit with my wife for the morning as her advocate, and as her companion.

Imagine, she volunteered her time to sit with Carole while still dealing with her own set of unknowns, her own set of fears, and her own set of physical and emotional traumas.

As close as I am with my wife, I still cannot know the pain and fear as well as someone who has experienced it firsthand. I was the lucky one, I was the comforter, I was the caregiver. These two women will be able to speak at such an intense and intimate level that not even my battle-weary soul would comprehend it.

I will say this a thousand times, and a thousand times more if I have to. They are the heroes. They are the wounded ones who kept fighting. Their fight is not over, but they will fight until it IS over. They never escape the battle, even temporarily. They either walk off the battlefield or are buried beneath it.

That room tomorrow will contain an awesome amount of reluctant courage. Until you have walked shoulder to shoulder with people like this, you just don't comprehend the utter bravery it requires of people who stand in such a profound solitude, fighting for their very lives against an invisible enemy hell-bent on destroying their bodies, their families and their futures.

Every country in the world has a military, and every military gives out medals for bravery.

There are no medals for these heroes, perhaps because they are fighting for their own lives, not the lives of comrades. But when you consider the husbands, the daughters, the sons, the parents, the friends that touch these lives, then perhaps the battle is not so selfish after all.

Is cancer really any less deadly than someone with a rifle? Isn't the battle the same, the bravery the same, the outcome the same?

I am not worthy of being in that room tomorrow. It is reserved for those who have faced this enemy eye to eye, and fought it hand to hand.

Neither will have earned the title 'survivor' by tomorrow, but with courage like that, it's just a matter of time.

F Words

April 17, 2011

My wife continues to heal and impress. I admit that there is a frustration in both of us, that progress is not the constant we hoped it would be. Good days are followed by bad days; days of optimism are followed by days of physical pain. No one who has been through these surgeries would be expected to be walking yet, but that's the problem. So few people have endured this gauntlet that no one is sure what progress is appropriate.

And that creates friction between the insurance company and the 'skilled' nursing facility. The insurance folks don't have a spreadsheet for this and the facility has no pre-approved therapy to get this patient back on her feet, so to speak. The insurance company has threatened to stop paying; the facility has argued that this is not your off-the-shelf patient. This is not news, it's just called 'Friday'.

In the grand scheme of things, this is not a game changer, but it is one more brick on the load for the caregiver. We are in the 'dog days' of recovery here. I can't report great, miraculous achievements, but I also cannot report significant setbacks. These are the middle miles of the marathon, these are the places where runners speak of 'hitting the wall' and transcending it, fighting through to a Zen place of rhythm and endurance.

We have no such place or pace. Every step is new, intentional, and wrought with its own costs and rewards.

She reacts to this by pushing through with guts, guts, and more guts.

I, unfortunately, don't respond so well.

No, I have more than my share of guts, in fact, they hang well over my belt buckle, but unlike my wife, my guts have no power to them.

I am fatigued. I am frustrated. I am fully engaged in this war but battle-weary. After all, I am human, and human is the last thing I need to be right now. I need to be rechargeable, reboot-able. All I know is that I need to be more than this, un-affected by where we are on the marathon.

I have just defined a machine. But that is what a caregiver becomes after the fatigue sets in and leaves. This fatigue is very human and physical, like dragging chains behind every step, like having muscles melt from your body.

At a time like this, you become a 'minute man'. I don't need to be tough every minute, just this minute. I don't need to feel anything every minute, just this minute.

A minute ago is ancient history; a minute from now is a century away. There is only this minute, this task, this problem to be solved.

Tomorrow we go to Stanford for a surgical follow up with the plastic surgeon. It's only been thirty days since my wife was literally cut in half. Will we get the permission to move to the next level of therapy?

I'll keep you posted, but until we go to the next level, we are stuck in the mud of rehabilitation. We may get to Stanford and back tomorrow, but unless we get the surgeon's blessing, we are in the same place we've been for at least another week.

I need to make the facility more responsive, the insurance company more patient, and the patient stronger.

And somehow, I have to find my soul again. I am too fatigued to have faith or feelings.

But considering the purpose of this battle, and the reward to the winner, perhaps I am just where I am supposed to be.

Fatigued, faithful...and still fighting.

I am sorry that there is no meaningful picture at the top of the post. I promise I will get around to it...when I get a minute.

Welcome to the Block, Homo-Erectus

April 19, 2011

It's another long frickin' story, but a critical med that Carole relies on to prevent nausea was unexpectedly stopped by the "skilled" nursing facility. It's a longer frickin' story, but I was the one who discovered it after going through the nurse's notes.

Why was I going through the nurse's notes? Because the ambulance crew that the insurance company paid $7,500 for to take us to Stanford, were EMTs, not Paramedics.

Why is that important? Because EMTs cannot give meds, according to California state law. I had to sign a consent form that I would dispense all her meds for the day trip to Stanford.

Let me get this right – a completely untrained spouse can dole out narcotics, but a trained EMT cannot. And, because this isn't silly enough, the nurses turned over a copy of all their notes to me to provide to the doctor at Stanford if needed, which I read on the trip up there.

And that's when I noticed that the Zofran nausea medicine had been discontinued on 4/15 with no explanation. And I speculated that this was the reason why my wife had been nauseous since Friday (the 15th).

How is an idiot like me, barely able to read a calendar, able to see that a critical med was discontinued? How was an idiot spouse like me able to see the change in my wife's condition since Friday, but trained, "skilled" nurses could not?

When my wife is nauseous, she cannot do her physical therapy or her occupational therapy. When she cannot do those things, the insurance company gets really grumpy and threatens not to pay. When they do that, spouses like me get called into the Admissions Director's office and informed that I need to find a place for my wife to reside in case this spat goes past this Thursday, otherwise I pay the full daily rate, plus pharmaceuticals.

On another note, did I mention that my friends think I have stress issues?

Here is the news that makes this all worth it – in spite of her not-insignificant level of pain and nausea, my wife got to the edge of the bed and stood up today. Yes, she relied on a walker and two spotters for balance, but she stood up on her own two uncertain feet.

Welcome to the block, Homo-Erectus. Guts like yours are always welcome. Inspiration like yours is hard-earned and rare, welcome.

Also welcome to the block, Bob, but you're passing through until you can match your spouse's guts.

At the moment, I am Homo-Idiot, dealing with Homo-Incompetent, forced to facilitate communication between Homo-Insurance and Homo-Skilled-Or-Not-Nursing.

There are tougher jobs in the world than mine, but if you're tough enough to stand after replacing critical parts of your spine with titanium thirty days after surgery, then you're tough enough under anyone's definition of tough.

I will be as tough as you someday, dear wife, but today Homo-Spouse-Erectus, the block is all yours.

Tonight, she healed me

April 20, 2011

The last couple of weeks have been brutal, even by recent standards. There are no enemies at the gate, but there are disappointments that pile up around us higher than the castle walls can defend. Recent history has been a constant story of promise and betrayal, all affecting my wife's recovery and comfort. I'll say this until my last breath, you can mess with me and get away with it, but if you mess with my wife...

It occurred to me recently that she and I have been involved with cancer and its betrayals and confusion for seven months now. It also occurred to me that even seven more months from now there are no guarantees that she will be walking and comfortable and back into life as most of us know it.

The grind has been stifling. There are days I feel there is no air to breathe anywhere on the planet, there are days I feel that everything has been a big, cosmic joke, that no one can be this unintentionally incompetent or clueless and still be considered a professional, or even an adult.

But I can find no joke, and I am certainly not laughing, at least not lately.

As well intentioned as some supportive but micro-managing people may be, as caring as some clueless professionals profess to be, as absent as some 'loyal' friends have become, we strive to fall forward daily with each step, but the steps are more and more costly.

Physically and emotionally, this is killing me.

Honestly, I really don't care how long I live; I just want it to be long enough to put her back together. (For the record, I know that sounds like an attention getting, look-at-me statement that underlines my suffering, but get over it. I'm never going to climb Everest, I'm never going to win a Grammy or a Pulitzer, and I'm not even going to be able to afford to retire. If this is my big win-or-go-home-moment, then I'll take it. Are doing any of those things really more valuable than this?)

Last night I could not sleep. Today I emailed work I would not be in.

Tonight, she healed me.

When I went to visit her she was comfortable and in good spirits. She knows me well enough to know I was hurting badly and, after some confessing conversation on my part, she invited me into bed.

Yes, bed. She slid over and after I took my shoes off, we hugged and cuddled for the first time in five weeks. Just her silent physical presence relieved me of the weight of it all, and my touch somehow comforted her, reassured her that this intimate support was still there, still hers. For a short time, life was returned to balance. For a short time, we were back before surgery, and separation, and titanium, and pain meds, and nurses, and strange empty beds to sleep in.

We talked of things we would do when she came home, like riding a bicycle built for two in the park, and renting an RV and hiding away from the world, and somehow enduring the kisses from three dogs who miss their mommy, and having our fickle cat once more cuddle in her arms. Somehow pain went away and life filled the void. The very planet realigned, the very cosmos ordered itself into the familiar pattern we knew, and her pulse once again made mine stronger.

Damn, it really is just this easy.

Eventually we were "caught" by a male nurse delivering a heating pad, but until then we were together, we were whole.

Tonight, a hole in my heart, a hole in my soul was filled, and I was complete again, even for a short time, but long enough to recharge my batteries and reload weapons.

This is the critical week where she demonstrates the strength and stubbornness I so intimately know into the progress we need to get out of custodial skilled nursing and into professional rehabilitation. This is the week we move through "nursing" into "rehab", and then "Home" into "Life".

Ironically, healing can be a two way street. Hopefully from this point forward, a busy two way street.

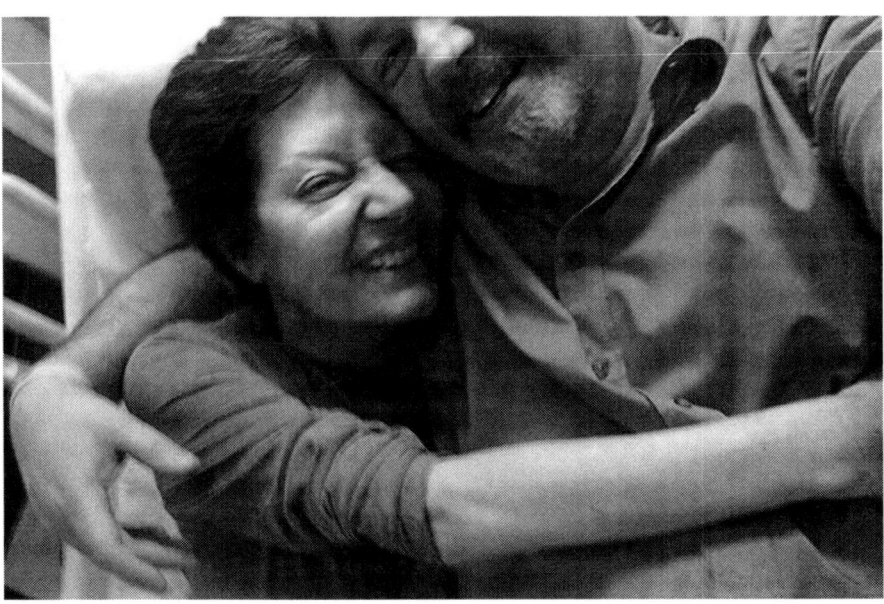

Stand Up, Stand Down

April 22, 2011

When will I ever learn?

I woke up today thinking that today was going to be an easy day. It was Good Friday, Carole's birthday and the company I work for was closing at noon. Perfect, work a half day and then go spend time with the birthday girl. Compared to what I've been through in the last seven months, this was a vacation day.

By 9:20, I had a voice mail from the "skilled" nursing facility. The insurance company decided it was time to move Carole to the physical rehabilitation hospital...TODAY.

Lock and load bald man, your day off is over, duty calls...

This turned into the classic 'hurry up and wait' military operation. Calls were made to the two best rehab hospitals in the area, but only one answered the phone. Luckily for us, it was our top choice hospital.

More calls were made; records were faxed, followed by a long, nervous wait. The hospital needed time to evaluate what they were given. In Carole's case, that's a lot of evaluating, since nothing in her medical records is cut and dried.

Since you're now waiting like we did, I'll take a minute here to report that the neurosurgeon called me yesterday and green-lighted my wife for all the physical therapy she can tolerate. This must have motivated the insurance company to move her up to the rehab hospital. This was all great news, but couldn't you guys have given us more notice?

As is typical in situations like this, adrenaline eventually waned and time slowed to a crawl. I started thinking "Please Lord, don't let this fall through...don't break her heart..."

During our waiting, the physical therapist arrived and I asked a favor of her, could she show me how to safely do the bed to wheelchair transfer, something we were not cleared to attempt until yesterday. She said yes and I ran down to the car and got Carole's wheelchair, the wheelchair I had been carrying since the day of surgery, hoping for a moment very much like this.

I have to admit that I was impressed by how effortlessly Carole stood up and was able to negotiate the transfer. With her nausea meds reinstated and her pain meds in balance she was much stronger than I expected. This is one tough girl...

After she got comfortable in her wheelchair, she started to explore her room, and after that she took a long look into the hall. A very few seconds after that, much like an otter silently dives below the waves, she was gone.

Down the hall she went, looking left and looking right. She looked out the hall window to the buildings across the street I take for granted on my trips to see her, but with fresh eyes.

After quickly soaking in the scene she made a u-turn and headed for the nurses station, picking up her pace, eyes wide like a child in Disneyland. By the time she was done, she had covered the entire floor, met nurses and residents she had never seen before, and peeked out of every window she could reach. It was like watching a little girl see her bedroom in a new house for the first time. The birthday girl tasted a freedom she hadn't known in five weeks, a birthday gift from a magnificent surgeon and a merciful God.

After we returned to the room, the time passed a little more easily as friends visited. One of our visitors was a former Marine friend of ours whom we had not seen in years. I don't know how the tyranny of daily life and not-so-insurmountable distance can create years between friends, especially friends of such quality, but this wrong was righted today.

At one point he asked me how tough the last few months had been. Both being veterans, it was easy for me to fall back into 'military-speak'. I answered that the intensity went from a "gentleman's war" to a very personal kind of battle, the kind of fight where you see the enemies eyes, feel their touch, and the heat of their breath. I used terms like 'fix bayonets' and 'hand-to-hand', I explained that there had been no strategy, no tactics, just survival by any means, the most basic and intense struggle in all of war, and all of nature.

I initially overlooked his reply, but later I would realize how much wisdom I had been gifted with.

At exactly 5:01 pm, after all of our cheerful visitors had left, and all our hopes were stretched to their max, my phone rang. It was the rehab hospital – she was in.

We both sat quietly on the bed, my arms around her and her head on my shoulder, and we just took it all in. In spite of the hard work ahead, we believed she had endured the worst.

She survived months of uncontrolled pain, months of uncertainty, weeks of waiting for a diagnosis, and even more weeks waiting for a drastic surgery to remove a mass the size of three of my fists. Add to this rebuilding her back with rods of titanium, the intensive care units, the 'skilled nursing', the seven hour ambulance rides and missing medications and you have a gauntlet few humans have ever endured.

As I looked at her, I realized that she was smiling like in the old days. I realized that she was not whole, but healing quickly. I realized that she was now safe, and unstoppable.

It's then that my friend's advice began to resonate through my head, and then my soul. His advice to me was simple – "it's time to stand down".

"Stand Down" means the danger has passed, the fight is over. This is when the weary emerge from their refuge into the carnage on the field. This is when the cold reality sets in that the losses are permanent, irreplaceable, irreversible.

Our irreversible losses are a portion of Carole's spine, a length of her bowel, seven months of her life and sight in her left eye.

In exchange for these losses we have a titanium sacrum, scars on front and back both measured in feet, hope that the cancer is gone forever, and twenty more years together.

Some warriors fight for their country, their comrades, or a cause. I was much, much luckier.

I fought for a soul simply worth fighting for. I fought for the woman I love. I fought to keep my promise — 'in sickness and health, until death do us part'.

Today, I am standing down.

Today, I am standing down because she is now strong and unstoppable. I am standing down because the fight is over, and I am content to pass into the echo of her success.

I am standing down because she can now stand up for herself.

The End.

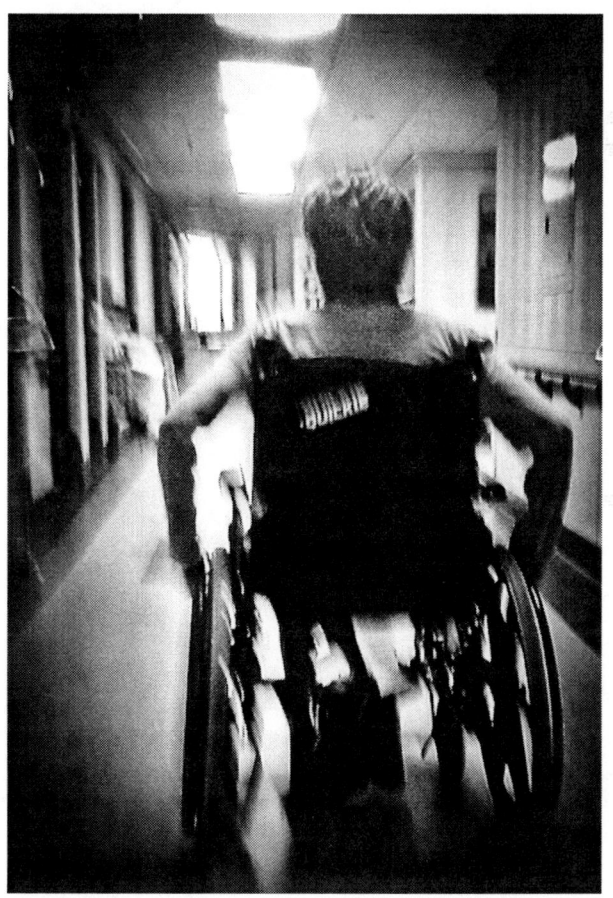

GRADUATION DAY

April 23, 2011

Upon entering her room I saw the same smile I left the night before. She was genuinely happy for the second a day in a row. It's only two days in a row, but they were very long in coming...

I had previously contacted the rehab hospital and they said they could accept her after 1 PM. This was great. I didn't want the waiting to wear on her any more than necessary and exhaust her.

Or me.

I did not sleep well last night. All I could think about was moving her to the rehab hospital of our choice, the rehab hospital we toured before surgery. This was an exceptional stroke of luck in my mind, and it made me as happy to transport her there as she was happy to be going.

After what seemed like a day in itself, we finally started the journey down the hall, down the elevator, and into our car. I was privileged to push her wheelchair and started quietly humming the song that high school bands play at graduation. After the first verse I decided, 'to hell with it' and starting humming loud enough so every one could hear. That triggered envious smiles from the residents, most of whom will never know this day, and satisfied smiles from the staff.

It was her moment, it was my wish come true, and it was a huge accomplishment for the both of us. From last Halloween until now, from the first symptoms to the last goodbye before surgery, from the moment it was all explained to us, this was the moment we had been focusing on.

Rehab is the last step before home.

Home is the first step in the rest of our lives.

This is where it starts.

Let's roll.

Once we arrived at the rehab hospital, it was like walking onto the bridge of the USS Enterprise. They were expecting us; someone had been assigned to transport and welcome her. There was a sense of value that the hospital was giving to the patient in the first few minutes, and it was soaked up gratefully by the patient and her spouse.

By the time my Mother-In-Law and I left, we were both breathing easier. My wife, and her daughter, was in her room and in her bed, and most importantly, in a place I trusted. There will be no need to ask volunteers to sit with her in shifts, because I trusted the professional ambiance the people and place projected.

Tomorrow is the first test. When I arrive, I will be acutely aware of my wife's level of pain and her level of comfort. Tomorrow, I am hoping is the first day I can start dropping my guard. Tomorrow, I hope that all my hopes are confirmed.

Tomorrow, hopefully, is the start of a challenging period that leads to a life filled with appreciation for the large and small miracles that surround everyone.

Today she graduated out of "skilled" nursing, but the day she comes home will be the day we both leave our previous lives behind and live a new life filled with understanding of just what suffering is, and just what "living" really means.

The Art of Survival

April 28, 2011

There are times when creativity seems to go dry, like a well in summer, but "artists" have a faith that the well will refill in time. This confidence is not driven by faith in wells, but faith that a "true artist's heart" would burst if creativity stopped completely.

Whether or not the heart inside of you, or me, belongs to an artist, is up to other people to judge. The sense that your heart will burst from not being emptied, from not being allowed to express itself is pure fact to those whose ribs contain such a heart.

And the idea that an artist "creates" is bogus on so many levels. True artists realize they are blessed by being mere pipelines, the conduit between the muses and the masses, much like the prophets of the Old Testament. Artists are not worthy of being called messengers, that is the work of angels. No, artists are merely pipelines buried beneath the surface of "reality".

And what is pumped through this pipeline is a need to show the masses how they appear while they are totally immersed and distracted by their own "culture".

Art forces comparison between how a culture appears from within and how that same culture is perceived from without. Art attempts to contrast the actions and ideals of a culture with the moral voice which whispers in the back of each person's mind. A person typically knows what is right, "people" can be manipulated to do anything, an artist intrinsically seeks the difference.

An artist only finds rest in truth, and only finds completeness of expression in absolutes, -absolute right and absolute wrong, absolute beauty and absolute repugnancy, – even though the art itself is often expressed in shades of gray.

The art of Carole's survival was certainly a work done in shades of gray, but it is an unusual work since it involved two artists. There were some very dark days and some very optimistic days, but each day throughout all of this had its own color, its own weight, its own individual truth depending on how our colors blended. Some days she was light and I was dark, some days we were almost the same shade, most days we were very different.

Taken singly, one day is almost identical to the previous day, but when you step back you can see how our individual shades formed a yet untitled mosaic of time and emotions.

Only the combination of two artist's hearts could create this work or survive this gauntlet, our strengths and weaknesses crested in a synergy greater than both of us; creating something indescribable in words, painful yet beautiful, and wholly unconquerable.

The well of our "creativity" will eventually refill, and as we step out of our culture of survival into the culture of the living, it will be with new absolute truths redefined by our struggle.

And throughout the life we have left together, we will often give pause to look at our bittersweet mosaic, now titled "The Art of Survival".

I Never Wanted A Tat

I never wanted a tattoo. Nope, wasn't even tempted in 50+ years.

I never wanted to see my spouse suffer pain, or have to work so hard to get around, or watch her struggle to see.

I never wanted to see her make a decision no human should ever have to make, a decision to sacrifice her ability to walk in exchange for staying alive.

I never imagined seeing her so compromised.

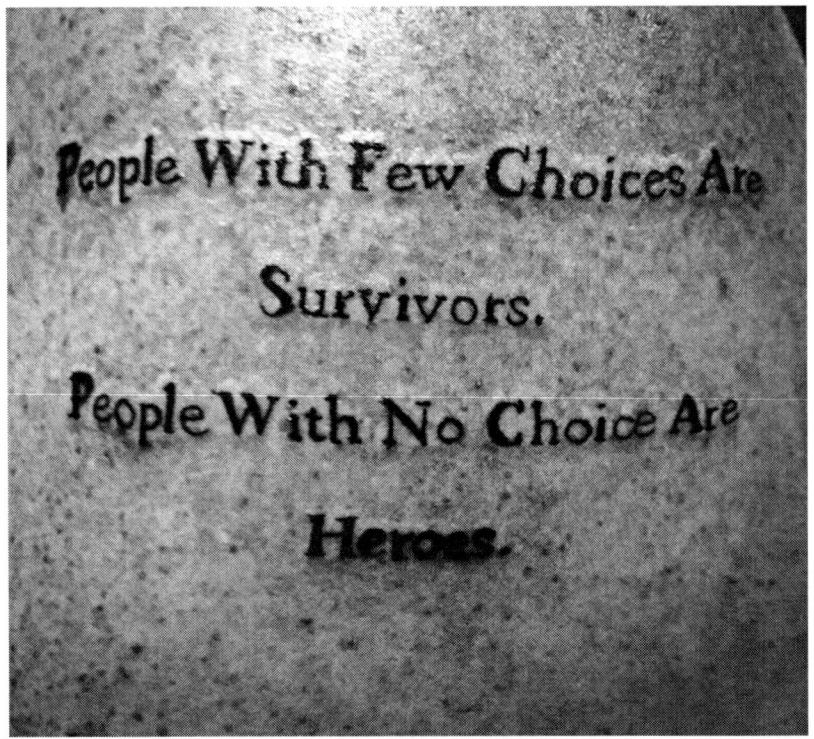

I also never thought I would see her so strong.
She's the hero.

Epilogue

There is so much more to this 'story'.

In total, from the day we left for the surgeries at Stanford through 'skilled nursing' and the physical rehab hospital until Carole returned back home was 52 days.

Since she has been home we are learning to deal with her physical rehabilitation, her sight loss, and my unemployment. The level of care Carole needed once she got home from one of the most dramatic and intense surgeries any human being has ever been forced to endure was greater than the patience of my former employer.

And today, October 12, 2011, the day before we planned to turn this manuscript in to the publisher, we got a call from Stanford. They want us to come in for a 'minor' surgery to remove suspicious growths from Carole's lung.

And with that, it all starts again...

Add Your Voice

Just because this book is done does not mean the struggle to care for our loved ones is.

I strongly encourage you to visit www.besidesthecancer.org and add your voice. You can tell everyone what you think about this book, you can ask for advice from other caregivers, you can vent at your frustrations with insurance companies or the medical system. Even if you just read the posts, the important thing to know is that you are not alone.

No one should be alone at a time like this, especially you, the one to whom so much responsibility falls. Care giving is a very heavy weight and it's best lifted by many people.

Let's lift each other up while we're at it.

Please Add Your Voice.

CPSIA information can be obtained at www.ICGtesting.com
Printed in the USA
LVOW081247080312

272173LV00002B/263/P